Lumbar Discography

Single Surgical Procedures 14

A Colour Atlas of

Lumbar Discography

C. Edmond Graham

Walter de Gruyter · Berlin · New York 1984

C. Edmond Graham, FRACS, FRCSE, FACS;
Visiting Orthopaedic Surgeon,
The Prince of Wales Hospital, Randwick, Sydney

Original Publishers: Wolfe Medical Publications Ltd., · London
Exclusive co-publishers for the Federal Republic of Germany and Austria:
Walter de Gruyter & Co., Genthiner Strasse 13, D-1000 Berlin 30. 1984.

Printed by Royal Smeets Offset b. v., Weert, Netherlands

Cover design: Rudolf Hübler

General Editor, Wolfe Surgical Atlases:
William F. Walker, DSc, ChM, FRCS (Eng.), FRCS (Edin.), FRS (Edin.)

CIP-Kurztitelaufnahme der Deutschen Bibliothek

Graham, C. Edmond:
A colour atlas of lumbar discography/
C. Edmond Graham. -
Berlin; New York: de Gruyter, 1984.
(Single surgical procedures; 14)
ISBN 3-11-010145-9
ISBN 3-11-010144-0 (Subskr.-Pr.)
NE: GT

Contents

Acknowledgements

The precise essentials of photography were skilfully provided by the well known Sydney photographer, Mr David Liddle, who prepared the transparencies. His relentless pursuit of excellence was as greatly appreciated as was his unflappable personality.

Julie Eichorn prepared all the diagrams with utmost care and thoroughness. Her artistic skills are plain to see.

The arduous secretarial work was performed uncomplainingly by Judy Turnbull who tolerated each 'change of mind' with good humour and great patience.

The proof reading was left in the capable hands of my wife, Dr Sian Graham.

I am deeply indebted to Dr Rodney J. Clark whose skill in the field of anaesthesia enabled these discograms to be performed without the patient feeling pain and yet with a pain response being elicited. Dr Clark was responsible also for the information provided in the paper regarding the premedication and analgesic agents used.

My thanks and gratitude go out also to the matron of Pacific Private Hospital and to her theatre staff who provided such an excellent service.

The Golden Fleece print (**1**) places me in the debt of the Art Gallery of New South Wales who gave me permission to reproduce it.

Introduction

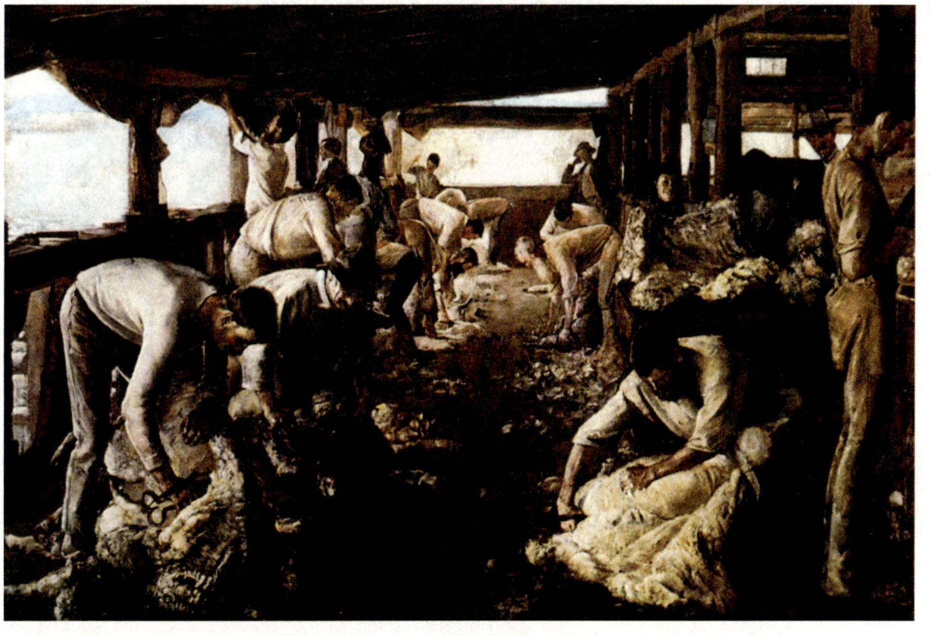
1

1 The flexed spines of the shearers. This scene by the artist Tom Roberts (and reproduced by courtesy of the Art Gallery of New South Wales) depicts the back breaking job of the Australian shearer. It is not surprising that the only constantly upright mammal in the world frequently emits the lament 'Oh, my aching back!'. It has been estimated that each year in the United States over 180,000 back sufferers submit to the surgeon's knife in the hope of curing or at least easing back pain and sciatica. Discography is a potent method of investigating such low back pain, and is defined as the introduction of radio opaque fluid into the nucleus pulposus for the purpose of identifying disc configuration and to demonstrate the functional status of the disc. There are two aspects of the procedure: firstly, the discogram itself (that is the osteograph with the radio opague material in the nucleus pulposus) and secondly, the patient's pain response to the injection into the disc.

The principal objective of discography is the diagnosing and locating of herniated discs in the lumbar spine and at the same time to attempt to reproduce the patient's back and/or leg pain, thus confirming the source of the discomfort. The accurate placing of a needle tip in the disc centre enables one to perform discography with its pain responses, volume and pressure assessments and gives us a picture of a herniated or normal disc. In addition, the well placed needle has therapeutic value because it permits the introduction of chemical agents such as chymopapain, chymodiactin, collagenase or cortisone into the nucleus pulposus in the hope that it will relieve back pain and sciatica.

In summary then, lumbar discography is performed as a precursor to intradiscal chemical therapy or as a precursor to laminectomy, disc excision and fusion. For the localisation of an offending disc pre-operatively it is more effective and more concise than a myelogram.

2 The anatomy of the disc and adjacent structures. The intervertebral disc is a 'cushion' which is situated between adjacent vertebrae. The two main components of the intervertebral disc are the annulus fibrosus or outer ring and the nucleus pulposus which occupies the centre of the ring. In effect, then, the annulus fibrosus surrounds the nucleus pulposus. It is attached to the chondral plate, both anterior and posterior longitudinal ligaments and to the body of the vertebrae. The annulus fibrosus gives the disc size, shape and tenacity. The nucleus pulposus is the semigelatinous centre of the disc. It is surrounded by the annulus and is the active portion of the disc, absorbing pressures, etc. The normal disc allows uniform transmission of forces. A herniated disc, otherwise known as a slipped disc, ruptured disc or prolapsed disc, is associated with the migration of the nucleus pulposus through a rent in the annulus fibrosus and in pressing upon the posterior longitudinal ligament causes back pain, or on a nerve root sciatica. Sciatica is a term used to describe pain over the course of the sciatic nerve, one of the major nerves in the lower limbs.

2

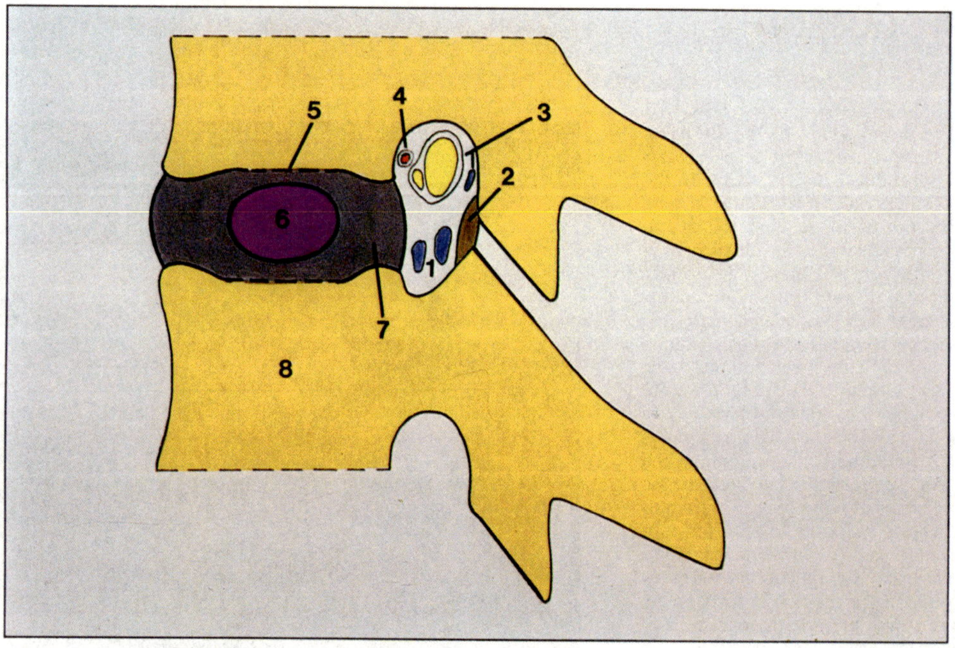

1 Intervertebral veins
2 Ligamentum flavum
3 Dorsal root ganglion and ventral spine root and radicular vein
4 Sinuvertebral nerve
5 Perforated chondral plate of vertebral body through which passes disc nutrients
6 Nucleus pulposus
7 Annulus fibrosus
8 Vertebral body

3

NEUROLEPT ANALGESIA

PAPAVERETUM (Omnopon) — *One Hour Pre. OP.*

DROPERIDOL — *I.V. 15 Minutes Pre. OP.*

DIAZEPAM = VALIUM — *I.V. Diluted*

THIOPENTONE — *Only for Deeper Sleep*

[FENTANYL (I.V.)]

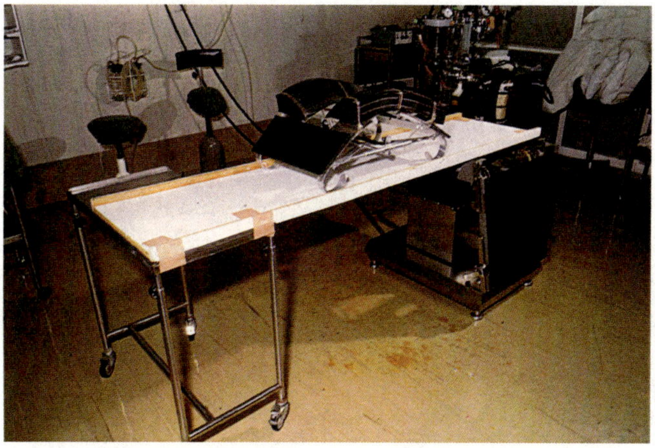

4

3 Drugs used to induce a degree of comfortable analgesia, without detracting from the pain reproduction. Since with lumbar discography we are endeavouring to reproduce the patient's back and/or leg pain, neurolept analgesia is used and this enables the patient to respond to a painful stimulus yet remain sufficiently sedated for it to be a reasonably comfortable procedure. This picture shows the drugs used to obtain this highly specialised type of analgesia anaesthesia. Papaveretum is used as an intramuscular injection 15 to 20 mg one hour before the procedure and this acts as a premedication – thus allaying anxiety and producing tranquillity. Droperidol 3 to 5 mg is administered intravenously 15 minutes before the procedure. Diazepam 6 to 15 mg is given intravenously diluted in the ratio of 10 mg per 5 ml. It is administered after the patient is placed in the prone position on the operating table. Thiopentone 100 to 200 mg is given intravenously on those rare occasions when the discomfort of the discographic procedure is too much for the patient and deeper sleep is deemed necessary. Some anaesthetists use Fentanyl as an additional analgesic. The blood pressure is monitored by the anaesthetist from the time the droperidol is given until full recovery is evident. Rarely is a patient unsuitable for the above procedure. In such cases a general anaesthetic using relaxants and endotracheal intubation is given.

4 The radio translucent discographic 'table' and pelvic rest situated above it. This strong plywood board measuring 2.5 cm in thickness, 194 cm in length and 50 cm in width, stretches from the operating table to an instrument table and is firmly attached to both with strapping. The plywood board is radio translucent and the width is such that the C arm of the image intensifier can be swung around to give anteroposterior and lateral pictures with one simple movement of the C arm. The pelvic rest, which is also radio translucent, is placed on the middle of the plywood board. Note that the edges of the plywood board stand proud in such a way that the pelvic rest cannot slip off the board during the positioning of the patient. Note that lumbar discography is carried out in the operating room or operating theatre under strict aseptic conditions. The pelvic rest is adjustable in both vertical and horizontal directions and this enables alterations to be made, depending on the size of the patient.

5

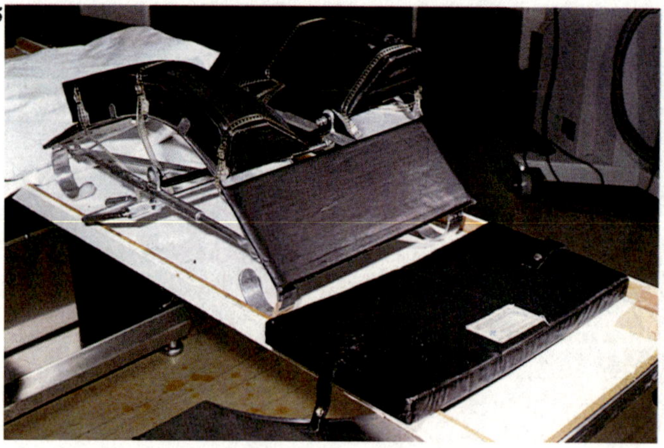

6

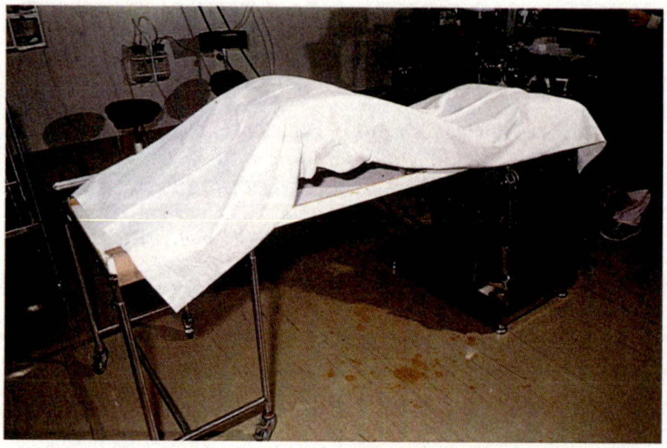

5 **Pelvic rest on table.** Another view of the plywood board and pelvic rest with additional knee cushioning seen on the right of the picture, and pillows for chest and head on the left.

6 **A white sheet covers pelvic rest and pillows and padding.** The bony parts are protected by pillows and padding and these are seen covered with a clean white sheet. The foot end is to the left and the head end to the right of the picture.

Transport of patient to discographic table

7
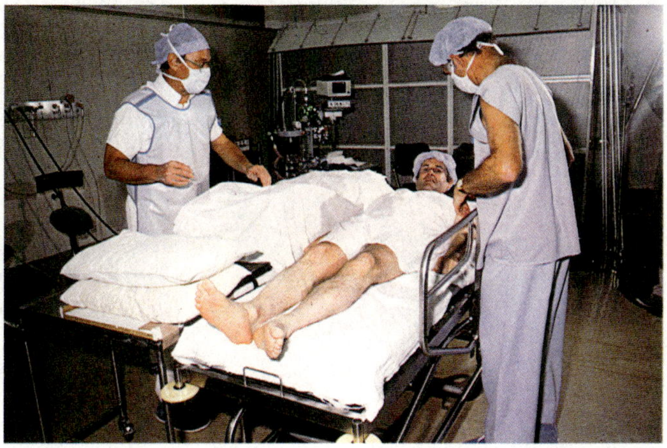

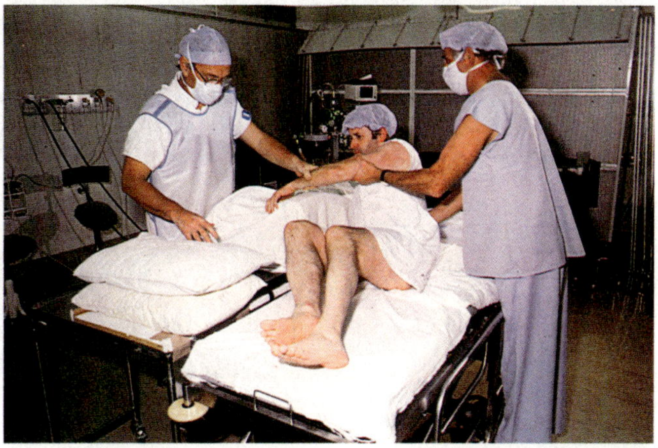
8

7 to 9 Transporting of patient from trolley to discographic table. In **7** we see the surgeon and the anaesthetist explaining to the patient, who is lying supine on the trolley, how he is to be mobilized into the prone position. In **8** the anaesthetist and surgeon are helping the patient from the trolley. In **9** the patient is seen kneeling on the soft pillow and beginning to lie on the pelvic rest.

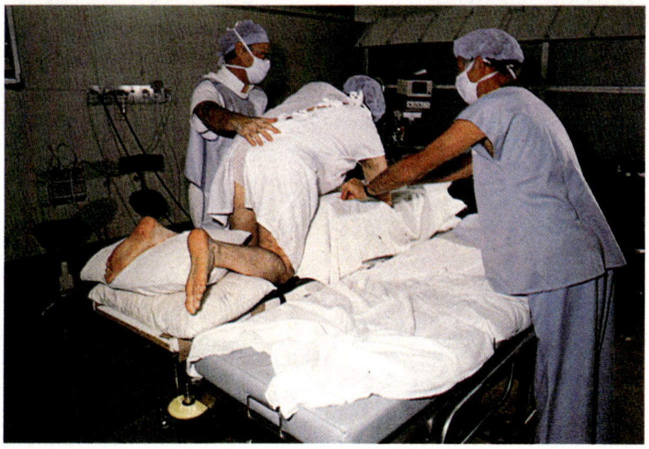
9

10 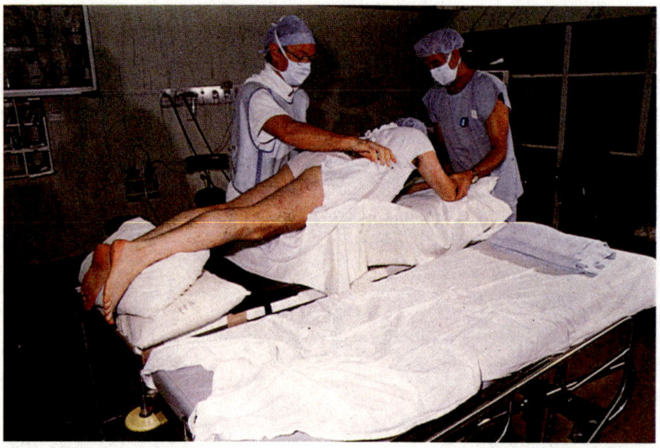 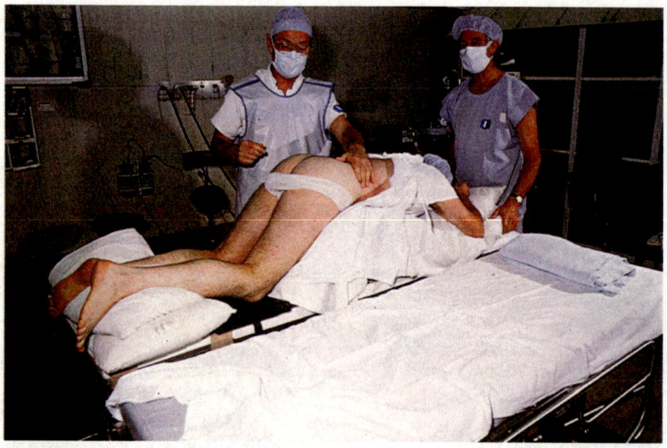 11

10 Patient has been placed on the pelvic rest in the prone position.

11 The feet are resting on a soft pillow, the knees are resting on a sponge and are semi-flexed. The hip joints are flexed and the pelvis is lying on the pelvic rest, which is covered with the white sheet, and the elbows and chest of the patient are comfortably placed on pillows with the anaesthetist making the final adjustments. The patient's lumbosacral region is flat and parallel with the floor. The radio translucent qualities of the plywood board and pelvic rest permit ready access of the C arm image intensifier to give an anteroposterior and lateral view of the disc area thus facilitating needle entry into the centre of the appropriate disc. Note that the bony parts are well padded and the ulna nerves protected from the pressure effects by sponge rubber.

12 The sedated prone patient has a sphygmomanometer cuff in situ and intravenous cannula in the vein on the back of the left hand. Note that the sphygmomanometer cuff on the left arm is to allow blood pressure readings to be obtained by the anaesthetist. This is essential, as the neurolept agents may drop the blood pressure suddenly. In the back of the hand is seen the intravenous cannula through which fluids such as valium for sedation or stimulant drugs such as adrenalin may be administered if necessary. In the rare event of anaphalactic shock taking place intravenous adrenalin, of course, is the drug of choice to control it. Some surgeons prefer to have the patient in the lateral position for this procedure of discography, but the author prefers to have the patient in the prone position.

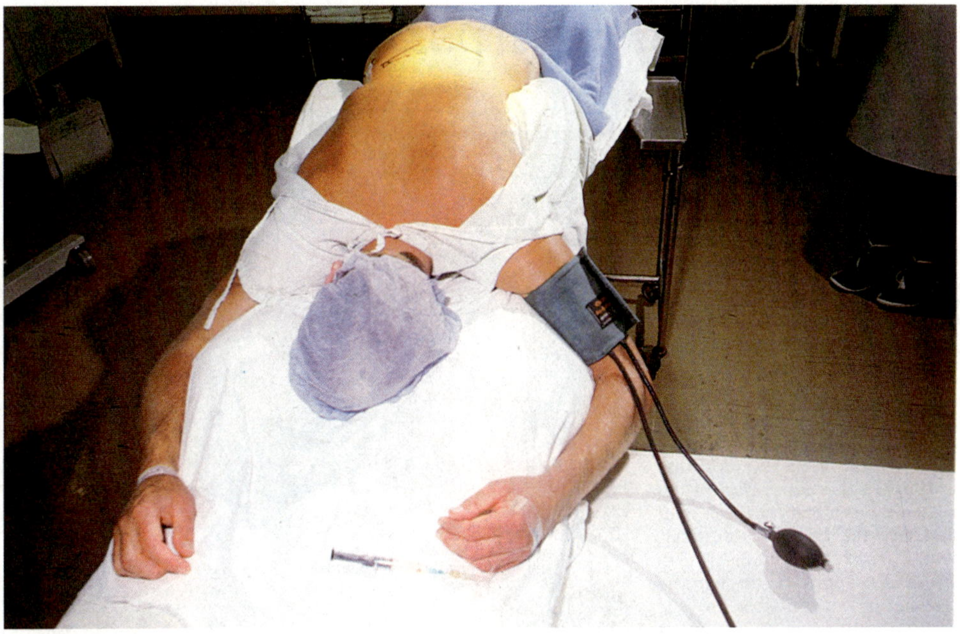

12

Identifying and marking important landmarks

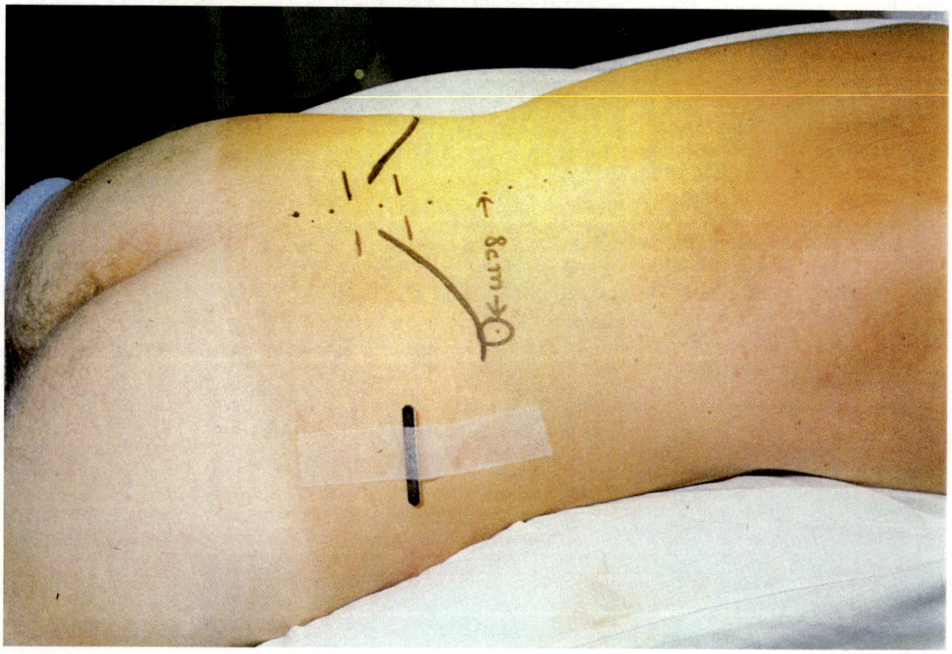

13

13 Identifying and marking important landmarks. Having made the patient comfortable a texta pencil is used to indicate important landmarks. The spinous processes have been marked with black dots in the midline and the spaces between the dots represent the interspinous gaps through which one may have to pass a needle if the lateral approach is unsuccessful. The right iliac crest has been marked with a texta pencil and a point 8 cm from the midline is circled. This circle represents the optimum point of entry for the preferred lateral approach for disc penetration. In the upper part of the picture one can see that for the sake of completeness the left iliac crest has also been marked. In about one case in 100 this lateral approach through the small circle is not possible, so the posterior interspinous approach is used. The vertically placed metal marker seen in the lower part of the picture and stuck to the patient with adhesive is put at approximately the L-5.S-1 level as seen on the lateral osteograph; this helps with the direction finding process for disc entry. Routinely the fourth and fifth lumbar discs are examined. When herniation of the third is suspected, it too is injected.

14 The hardware required for lumbar discography. From left to right on the green sterile cloth may be seen a kidney dish that contains a bowl of iodine or betadine and a sponge holding forceps with several raytec swabs. To the right of the kidney dish is a 25 ml syringe containing 20 ml of one per cent xylocaine. To the right of the 25 ml syringe are four lumbar discogram needles. These are 6 inches in length and are 18 gauge. To the right of the four lumbar discogram needles are the two needles used for the posterior approach that might have to be utilised when the lateral approach is not possible. The shorter needle is two inches long and is 18 gauge and through this is passed a 22 gauge 4½ inch long needle for penetration of the annulus. To the right of those needles is seen a 5 ml syringe containing Conray 280 and to the right of that is the small 2 ml syringe containing hydrocortisone or enzyme if it is to be used. The Conray 280 is the water soluble radio-opaque medium that is used to delineate the disc centre.

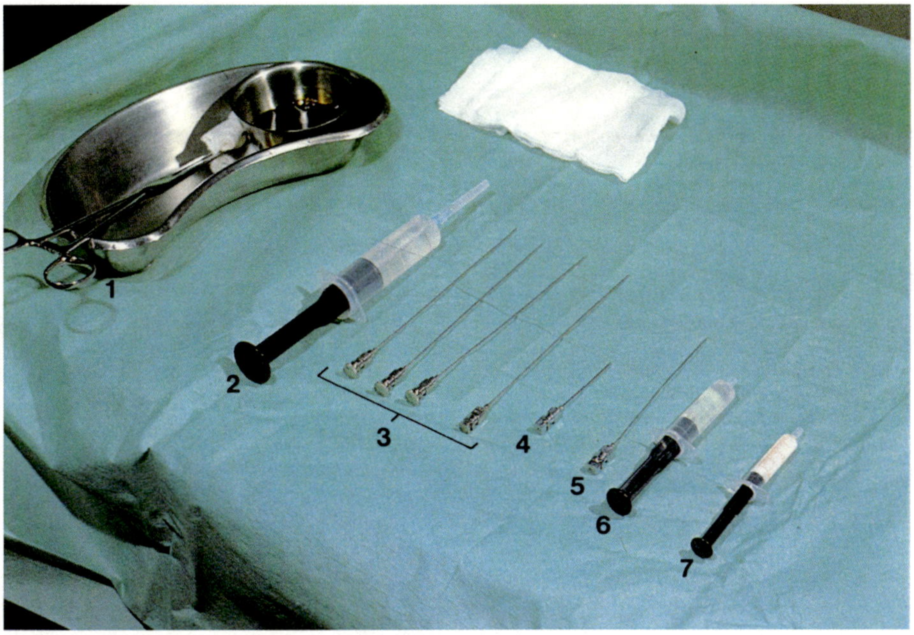

14

1 Kidney dish that contains a bowl of Iodine or Betadine and a sponge holding forceps with several Ratex swabs.
2 25 ml syringe containing 20 ml of one percent of xylocaine.
3 Four lumbar discogram needles 6 inches in length and of 18 gauge.
4 Two-inch long 18 gauge discogram needles that are used for the posterior approach that might have to be utilised when the lateral approach is not possible.
5 Four-and-a-half-inch long 22 guage needles used for the posterior approach and to be passed through the 18 gauge needles.
6 Five ml syringe containing Conray 280.
7 Two ml syringe containing either hydrocortisone or the enzyme chymopapain.

Three-needle approach

15 The three-needle approach to the lumbar discs. The lateral extradural approach is used because it avoids the transgression of the spinal canal and the puncture of the vulnerable posterior part ol the annulus. The structures seen in this picture include the posterior needle, the posterolateral needle, and the lateral needle; we can see the fourth lumbar nerve and the 5th lumbar vertebra. The interverte-bral disc is shown as well as the inferior vena cava and the abdominal aorta.

15

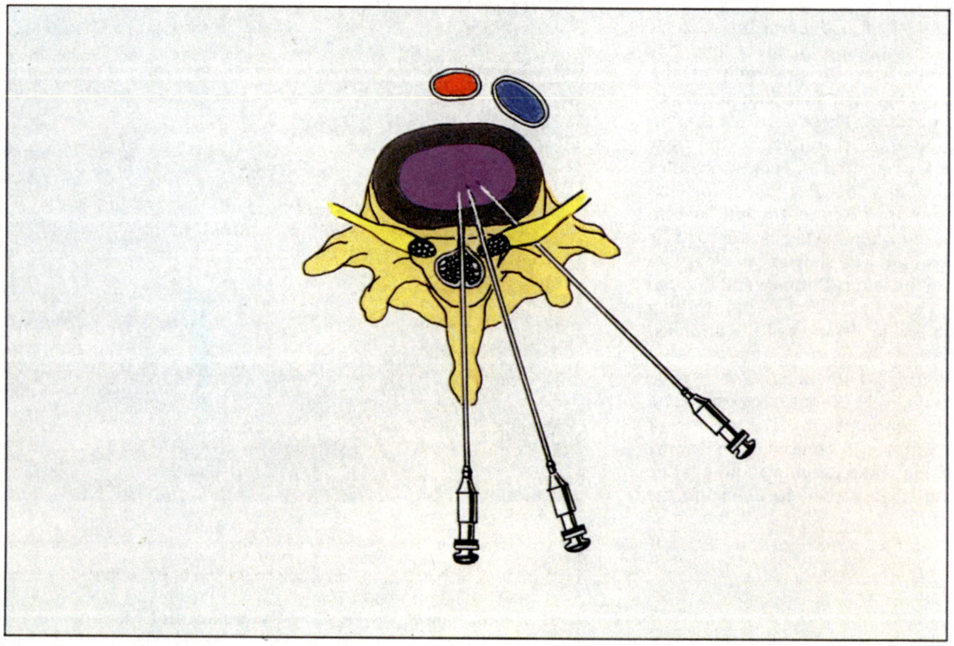

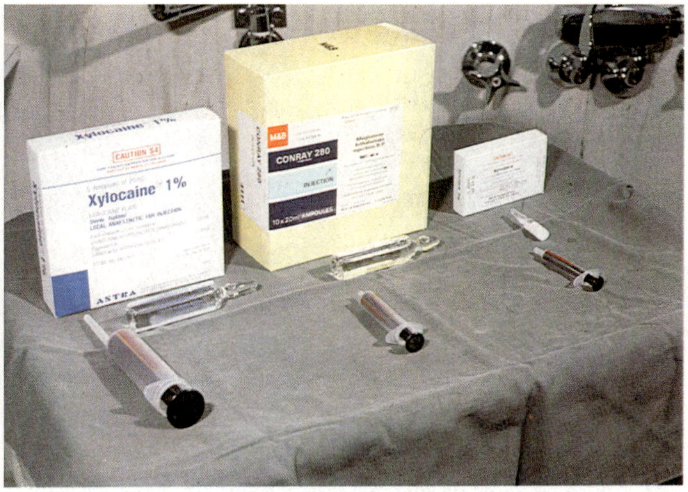

16 The drugs used for lumbar discography. Here we see the xylocaine one per cent ready for drawing up in a 25 ml syringe and in the middle of the picture the Conray 280. To the right is hydrocortisone acetate that is sometimes used therapeutically in the treatment of backache.

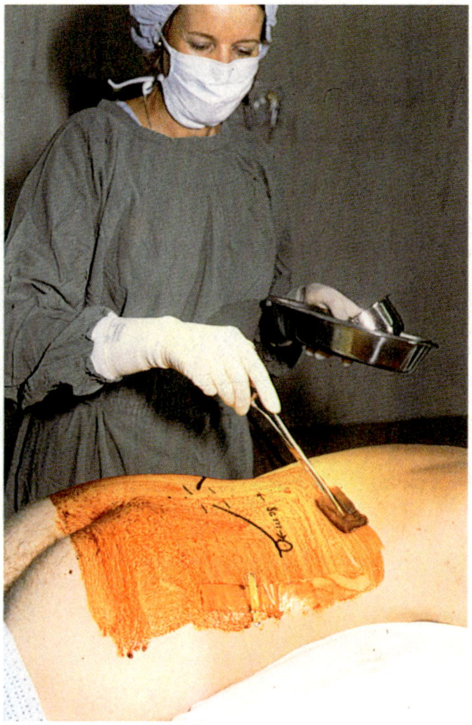
17

17 Skin preparation. After the surgeon has marked the area the theatre sister then thoroughly cleanses the skin with an antiseptic solution. Note that the area of cleansing is quite large and that the theatre sister is capped, gowned and gloved for this procedure, as is the surgeon.

18

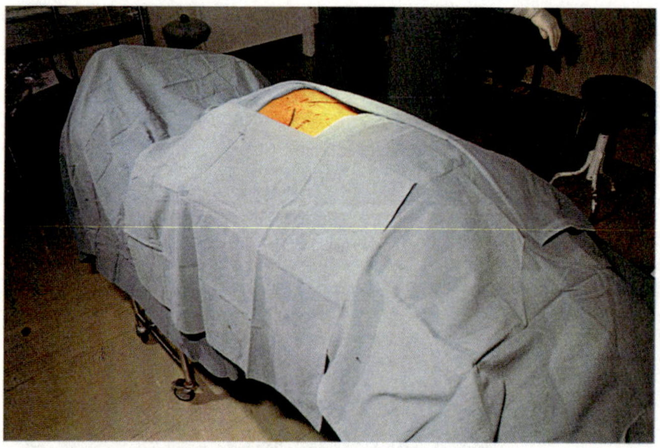

1

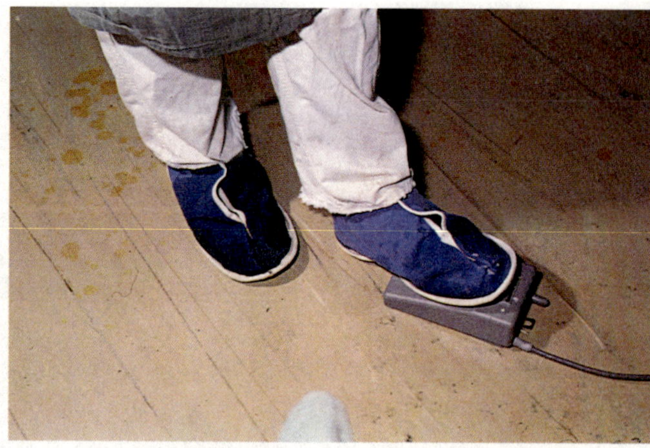

18 Draping the patient. The four green drapes have been applied in such a way that the area for needle approach has been left exposed.

19 Operating the image intensifier. The surgeon is operating the button by foot for the image intensifier to give him an instant picture on the television screen, thus aiding in the direction finding of the needles. It is more efficient for the surgeon to operate the image intensifier than for the radiographer, because he can move his hands from the field of irradiation a second or so before he irradiates the area. It is essential that a personal monitoring film be worn by the surgeon if he is a regular discographer; this monitor should be worn either under the leaden apron or on the forearm or in both places so that an assessment can be made at three-monthly intervals to assess irradiation risk. Note also that everybody in the room wears a leaden apron to protect their body from irradiation.

Anatomy of lumbar discography

20 The anatomy of lumbar discography. This colourful diagram indicates the significant anatomical structures of which the discographer should be aware, and represents a cross section at L-5.S-1 disc level. The following are the significant structures:

1a The local anaesthetic needle is seen penetrating the skin and lumbar fascia at a point 8 cm to the right of the midline
2 The skin
3 The lumbar fascia
4 The sacro spinalis muscle
5 Quadratus lumborum muscle
6 Psoas muscle
7 Spinal nerve
8 Transverse process
9 Lamina
10 Spinous process
11 Dural sac housing the cauda equina
12 L-5.S-1 intervertebral disc
13 Iliac vessels
14 Peritoneum
15 Ileum (small bowel)

20

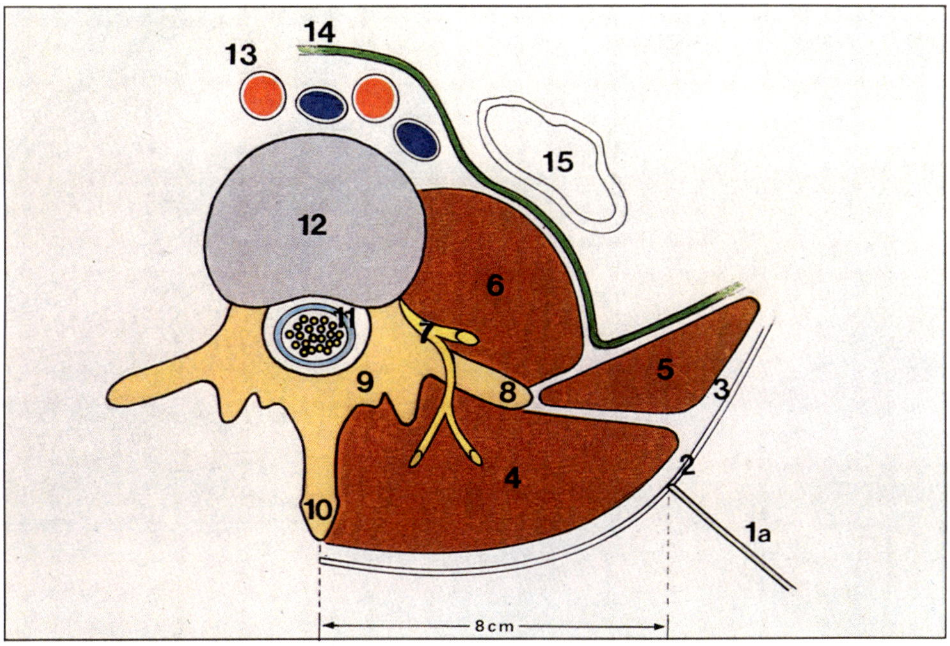

21 Introduction of the 18 gauge needle. The 18 gauge discogram needle is passed 2 to 3 cm through the anaesthetised skin and lumbar fascia and sacro spinalis muscle. A touch on the foot switch by the surgeon gives him an instant picture, thus indicating needle direction.

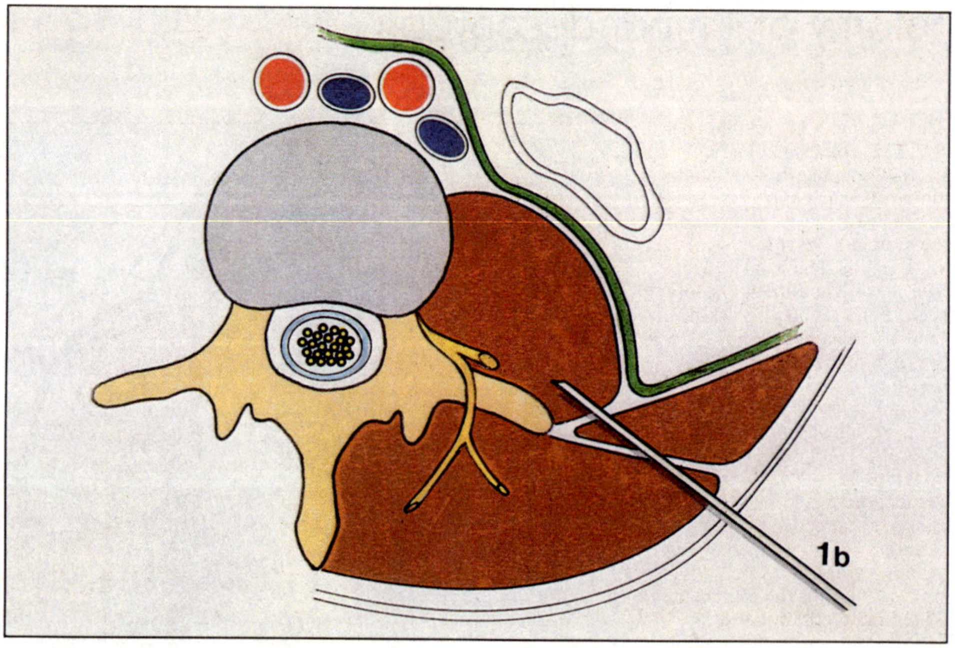

21

22 Further needle progression to transverse process level and beyond. Having passed adjacent to the transverse process the needle point safely traverses the psoas muscle to reach the annulus fibrosus at lumbosacral disc level. At this point local anaesthetic is injected into the annular area to prevent pain on disc penetration.

22

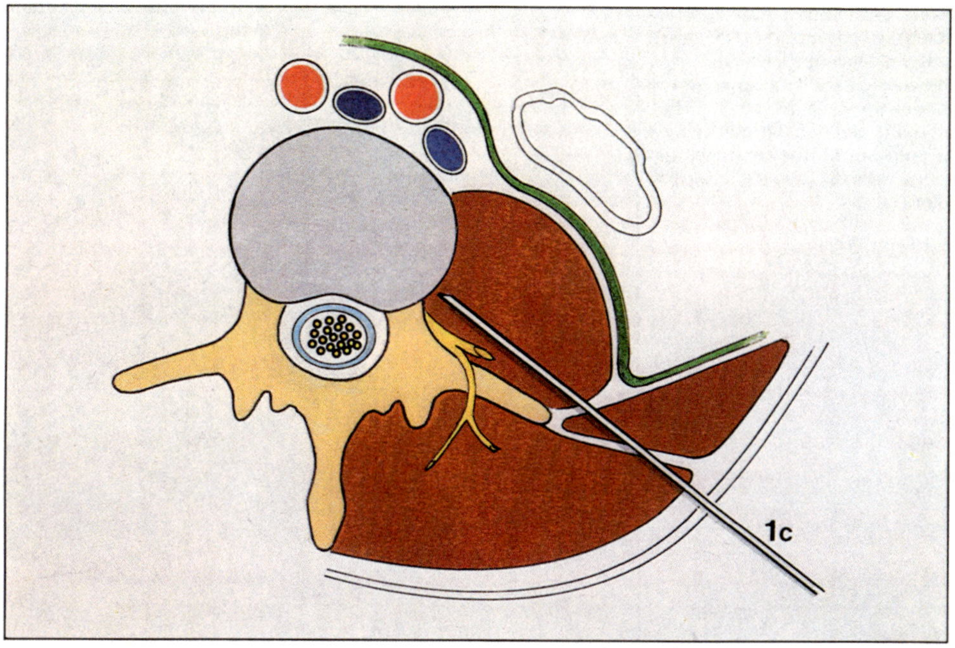

23 Needle advanced to disc centre. The needle is advanced to the disc centre after a delay of a few minutes to allow the local anaesthetic adjacent to the annulus to have its effect. The position of the end of the needle in the nucleus pulposus (**16**) is confirmed in two planes with the aid of the image intensifier.

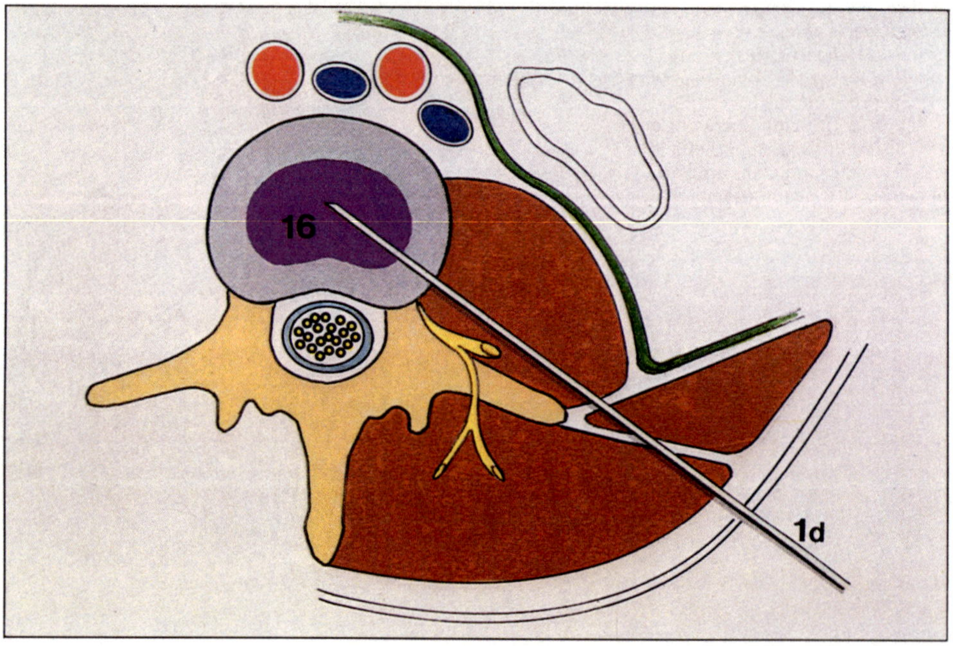

23

24a Needle too superficial. If the needle is placed too superficial or posterior then it might penetrate the lamina as seen here or transgress the dural sac, thus entering the subarachnoid space.

24b Needle too deep. A needle too deep or anterior could penetrate the bowel or a major vessel. Should the surgeon then unwittingly withdraw the needle from the bowel and then introduce it into the disc centre, the nucleus pulposus could be inoculated with E. Coli, thus producing a discitis.

24

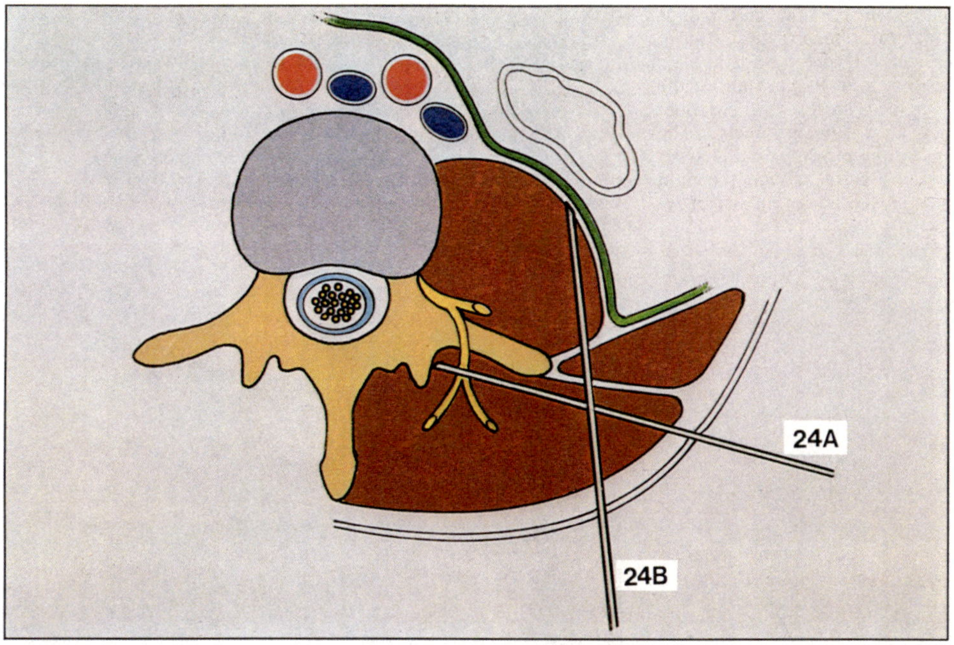

25 Infiltration of skin and muscle layers with local anaesthetic. 20 ml of one per cent xylocaine is being injected into the skin 8 cm to the right of the midline at iliac crest level. The right iliac crest area is being injected. The head end of the patient is in the lower part of the picture and on the right may be seen the image intensifier receiving arm.

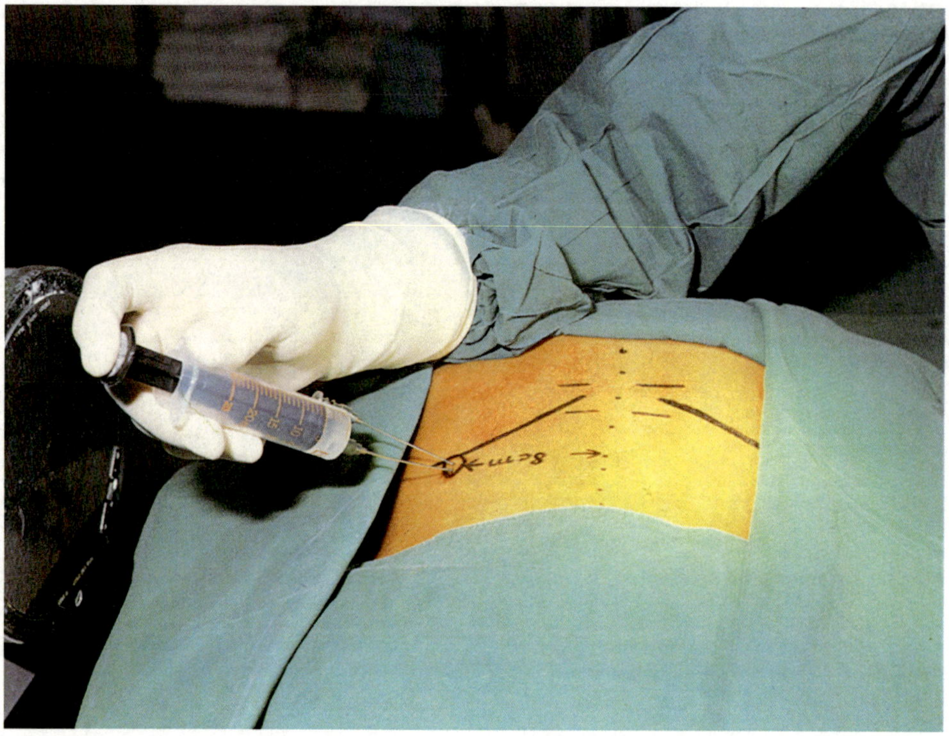

25

26 Directing the lateral needles as far as, but not into, the annulus. After a delay of two or three minutes or so to enable the xylocaine to have its effect, an 18 gauge six inch long needle is directed toward the appropriate lumbar disc. In this picture the 18 gauge needle has been inserted down to, but not through, the annulus. For entry into the L-4-5 disc the needle is directed in an antero medial direction 30 to 60 degrees to the horizontal and for the L-5.S-1 disc it is directed an additional 30 to 45 degrees caudally. Several readjustments may have to be made before the annulus of the two discs is reached and each time the needle is redirected, of course, the image intensifier button is operated for half a second or so to assist direction finding.

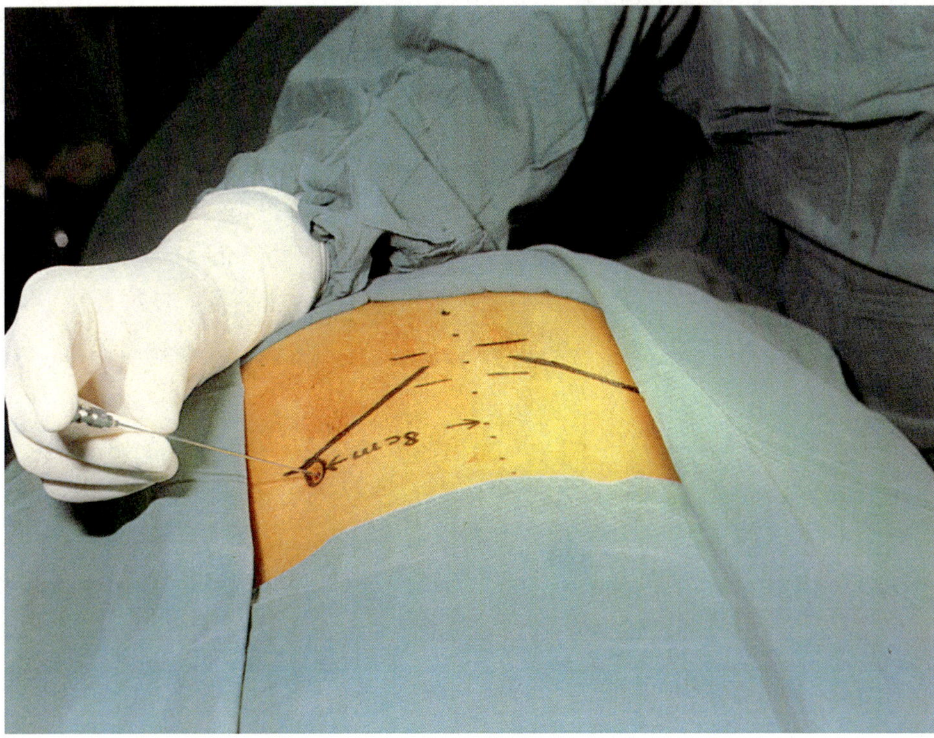

26

27 Needle direction. This picture taken across the patient's buttocks from buttock to head indicates needle direction and the needles are seen between 30 and 60 degrees to the horizontal. The blue dome is the cap covering the patient's head.

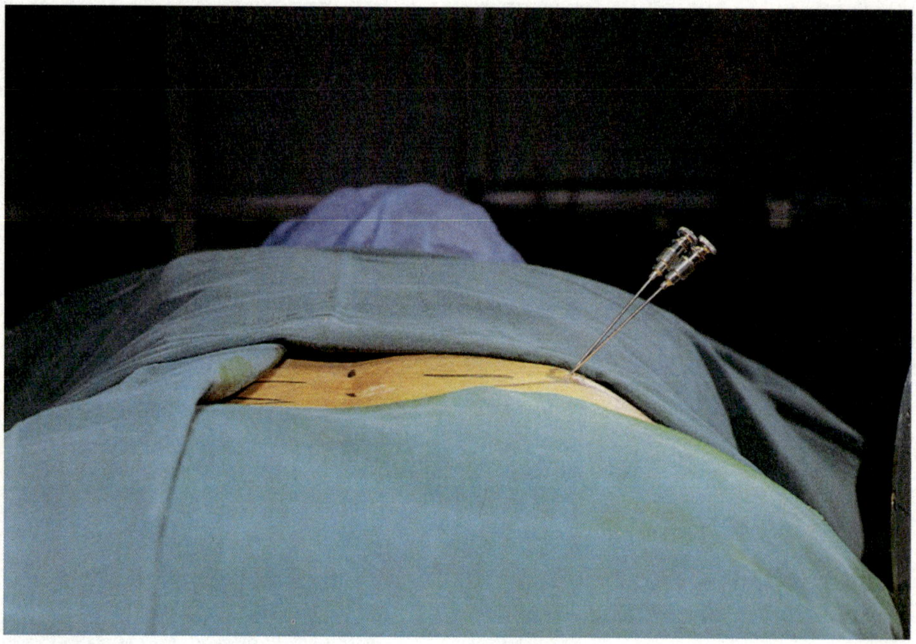

27

28 Needle direction. This picture taken from vertical position above the patient indicates the L-4-5 disc being penetrated by the horizontally placed needle, whereas the L-5.S-1 disc is penetrated by a needle that is manifesting an additional 30 degrees in a caudal direction. The upper needle, in the picture, is the caudally directed L-5.S-2 needle.

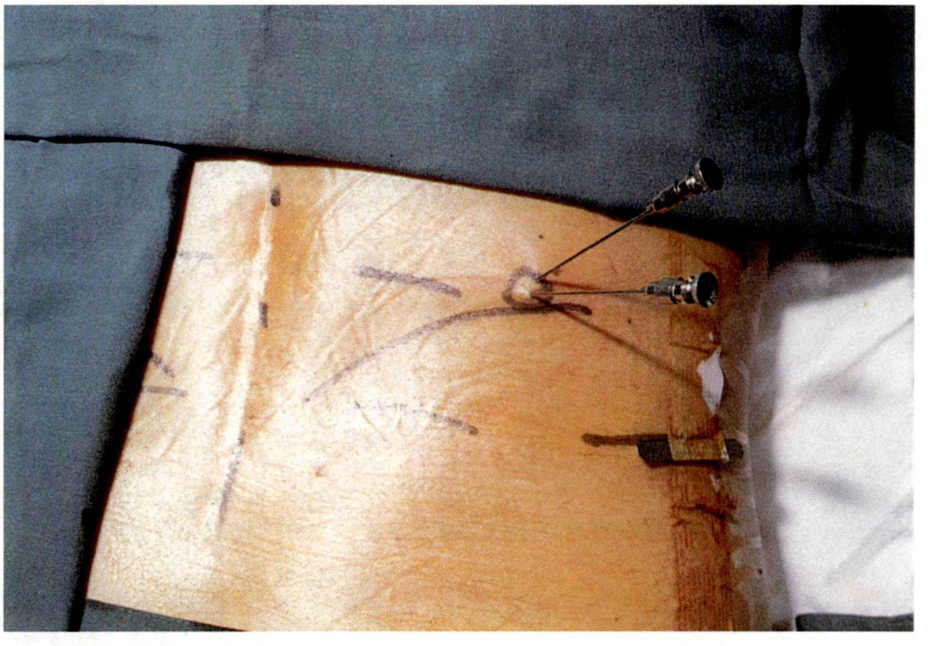

28

29 Needle points at the edge of the annulus at L-4-5 and L-5.S-1 levels. This osteograph shows needle placement. The needles have been pushed as far as, but not into, the annulus fibrosus at L-4-5 and L-5.S-1 levels. Since the spinal nerves are adjacent to the annulus at this point and since also the annulus itself may be painful on penetration, 3 ml of xylocaine are administered at each level and the procedure delayed for two or three minutes to enable the local anaesthetic to have its effect.

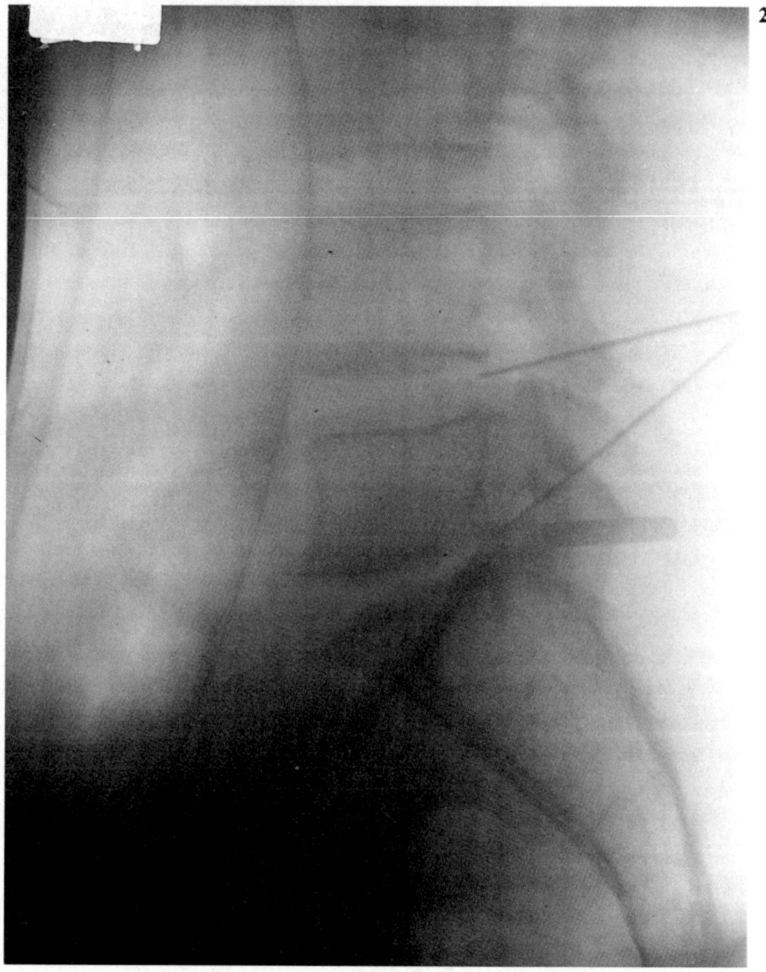

29

Annular infiltration with xylocaine

30 Annular infiltration with xylocaine before final penetration of the two discs by the needle.

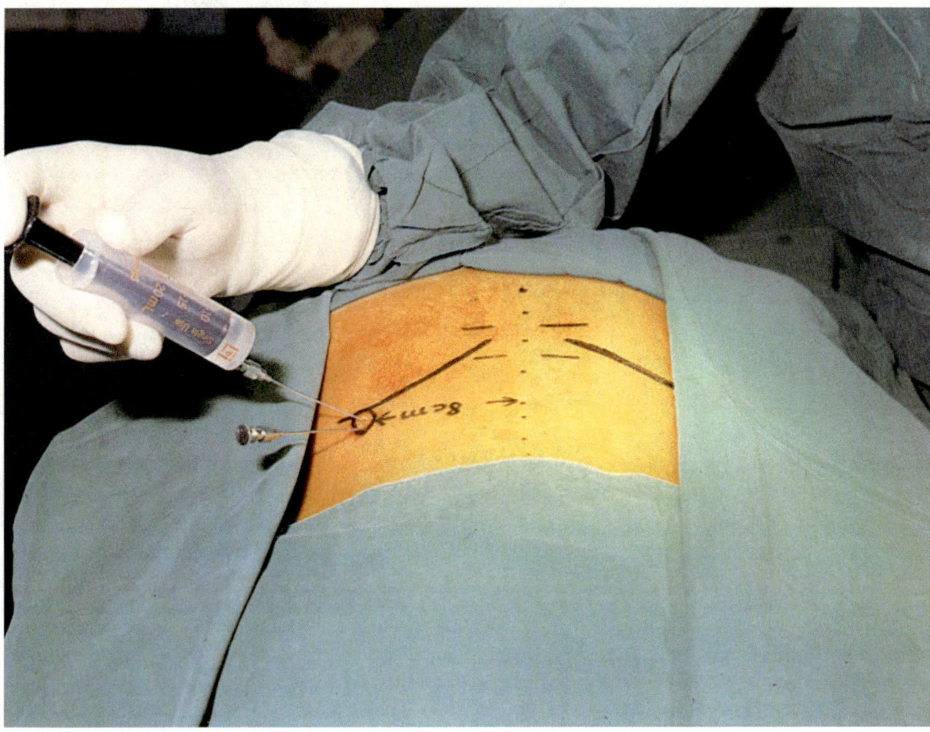

30

31 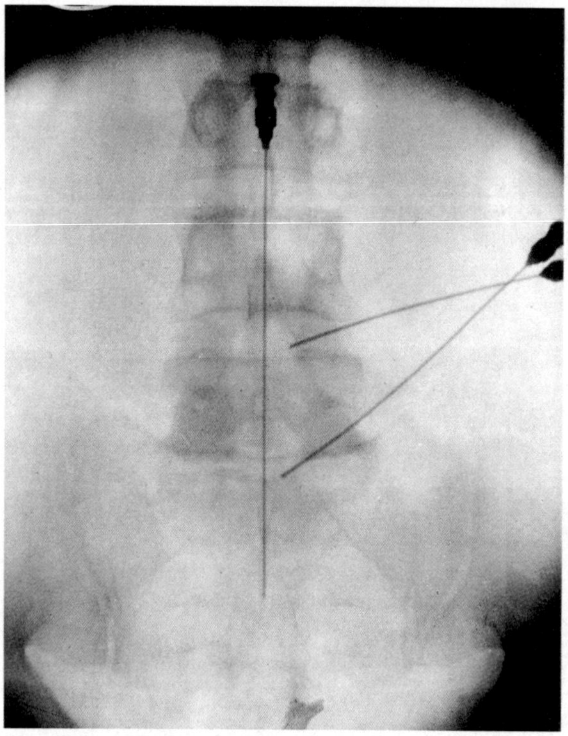

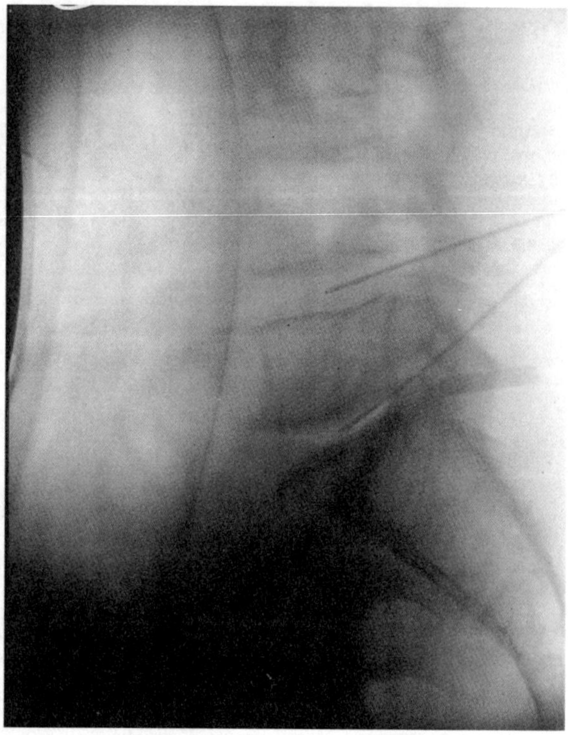 32

31 Anteroposterior osteograph showing that the needles have been driven almost to the midline and are virtually in the centre of the discs L-4-5 and L-5.S-1. The midline needle is simply placed there to make it easier to locate the midline, and is placed on the patient's back alongside the spinous processes before the osteograph is taken.

32 Needle placement. This osteograph shows the lateral view with two well placed needles, one at L-4-5 and the other at L-5.S-1. Some surgeons prefer to penetrate the annulus with a longer, thinner, 24 gauge needle that has been passed through the centre of the thicker needle whose tip is left to lie immediately outside the annulus fibrosus. It is the author's opinion, however, that the 18 gauge needle going in through the lateral approach does no harm to the annulus.

33 Infiltration of the skin with xylocaine in the midline in preparation for a posterior approach. The posterior interspinous area is being infiltrated with xylocaine because the surgeon was unable to place a lateral needle into the L-5.S-1 disc. There is one lateral needle in situ and the injection taking place is that of xylocaine being introduced between the L-5 and S-1 spinous processes in the midline. In exceptional circumstances this posterior approach is used when penetration of the annulus is not possible by the lateral approach due to the presence of a high iliac crest or large transverse process.

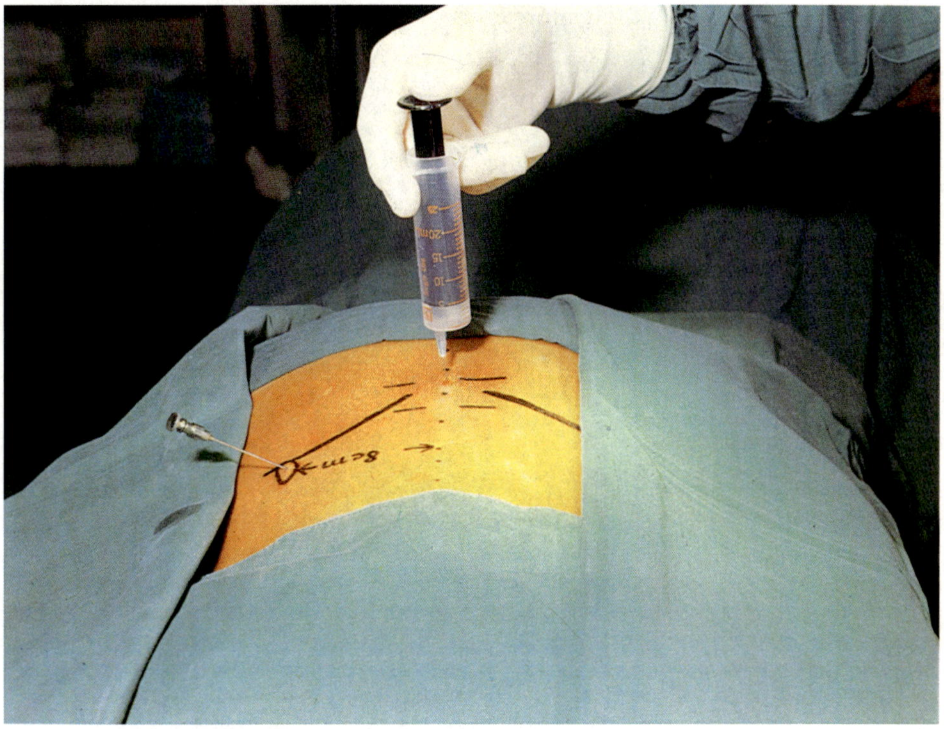

33

34 Placement of posterior needle in the midline following local anaesthetic infiltration. The needle is a two inch long 18 gauge, directed vertically through the inter spinous ligaments. It passes down to the dural sac but does not enter it. When it is seen radiologically to be in the correct direction for disc penetration a 4½ inch long 22 gauge needle is passed through the 18 gauge needle into the intervertebral disc. The image intensifier gives us confirmatory pictures in two planes that the needle end is centrally placed in the disc or discs. The disadvantage of this approach is that the needle penetrates the dural sac, thus creating the slight risk of headaches and meningismus postoperatively, and the slight risk of injury to one of the nerve roots that constitute the cauda equina. The laterally placed needle in this picture does not have that complication because it bypasses the dural sac.

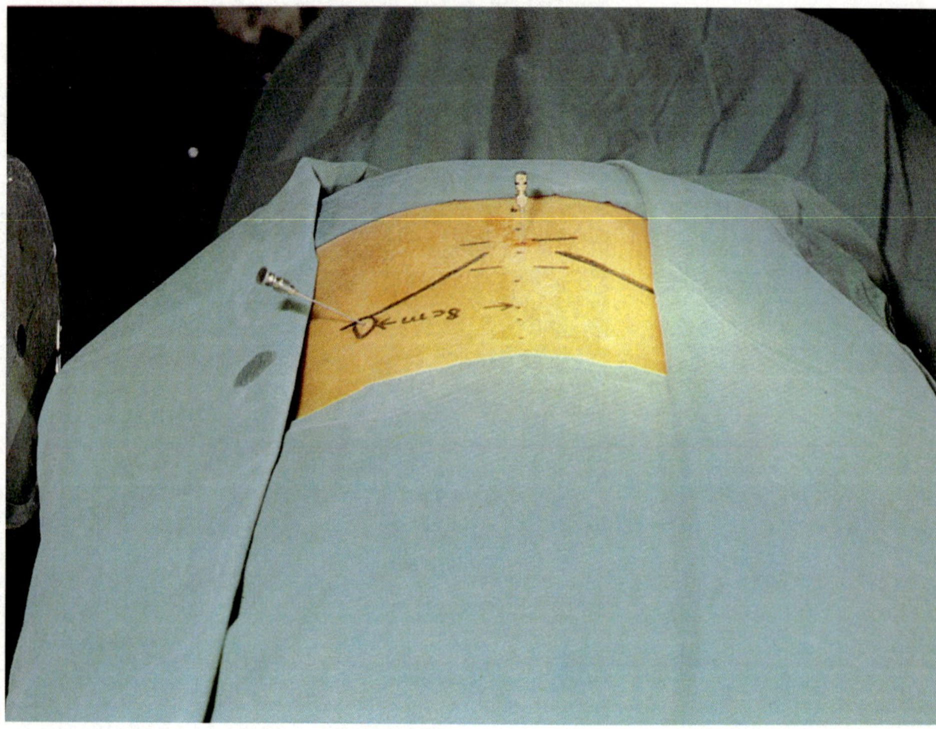

34

35

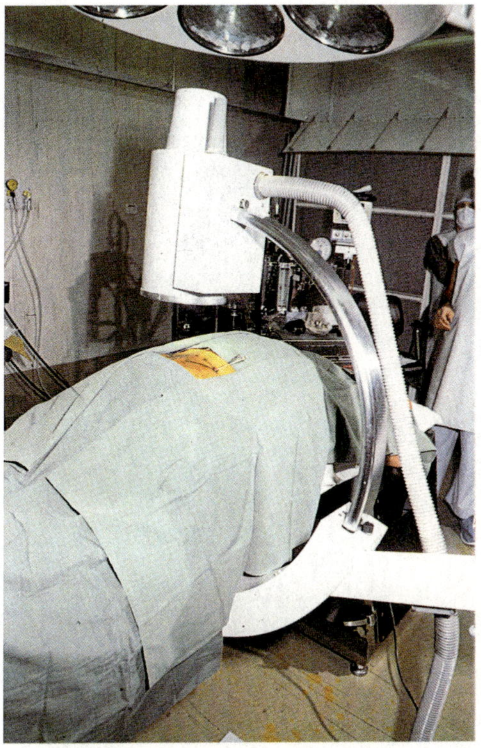

36

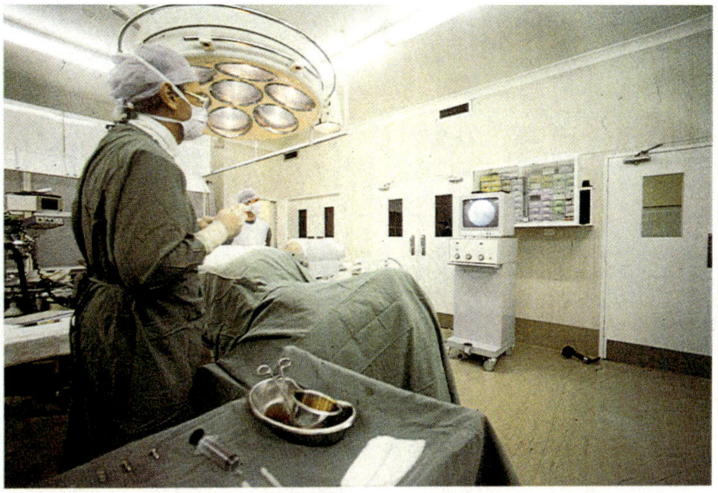

36 Placement of image intensifier screen. The viewing box of the image intensifier is situated in such a way that the surgeon can instantly see the position of the needles by depressing the foot button. Note the proximity of the TV monitor to the surgeon's field of vision.

35 Operating the image intensifier for anteroposterior view of disc and needles. The C arm of the image intensifier occupies a vertical position in this picture above the patient's lumbar spine and we are now able to obtain an anteroposterior picture to confirm the position of the needle tip.

Injection of contrast

37 Injection of contrast Conray 280 into the disc centres via the lateral approach. Injection of contrast medium. The well placed laterally directed needle is having Conray injected into it and the usual volume taken is 1 ml. The normal disc with an intact annulus will take 1 ml of Conray and the plunger of the syringe manifests considerable back pressure, thus indicating an intact annulus.

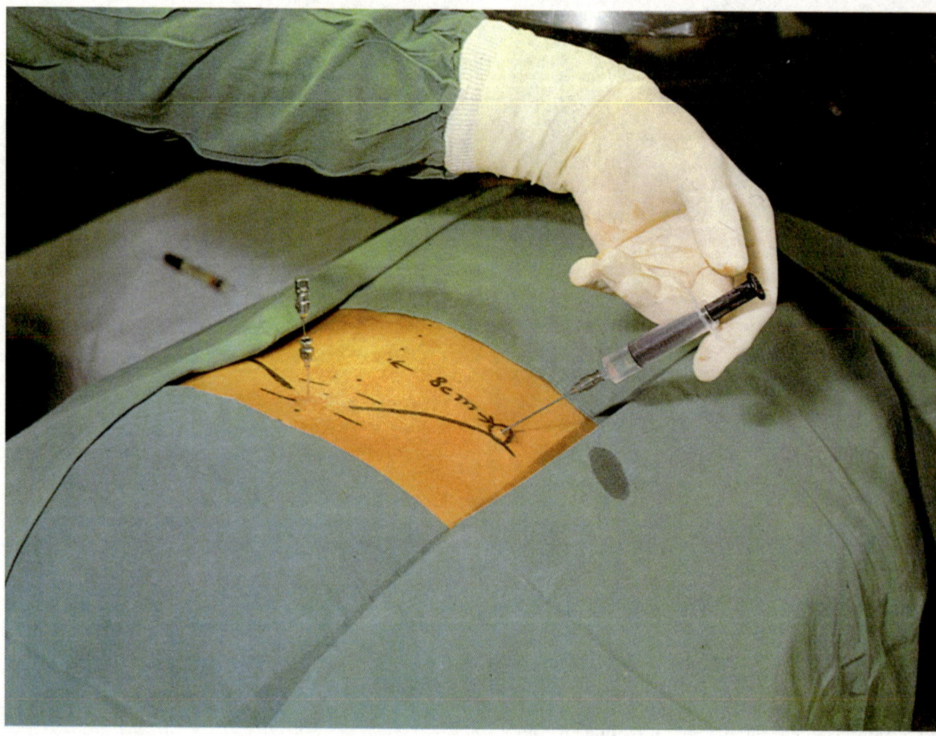

37

38 Injection of contrast Conray 280 into the disc centres via the posterior route. Conray is being injected through the less desirable posterior route into the L-5.S-1 disc because the surgeon was unable to gain entry into the L-5.S-1 disc through the lateral approach. The pain response and volume of the disc can be as readily measured with this approach as it can with the lateral approach.

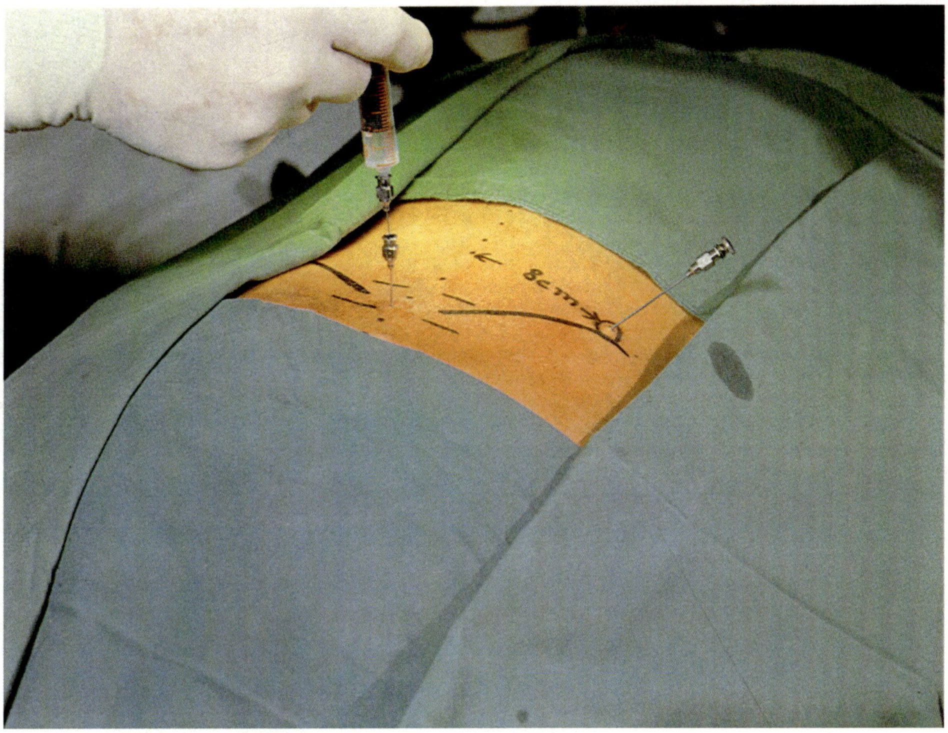

38

Patient interrogation

39 Patient interrogation. The anaesthetist is seen interrogating the patient regarding pain response during the process of injecting Conray 280. The filling of a normal disc with Conray 280 is a painless procedure, whereas injection of a symptomatic herniated disc can be extremely painful. The surgeon therefore injects 0.25 ml of Conray at any given time and asks the patient: *'Does this injection reproduce the pain that you have had before, in the back or leg?'* If pain is recorded it is instantly relievable by injection of xylocaine through the appropriate needle. The anaesthetist asks the patient if there is discomfort in the back, buttock or leg and if so whether it is similar in quality and distribution (same leg) as the pain the patient has had since his symptoms began. These enquiries regarding pain response are sought on each occasion that a disc is injected with Conray.

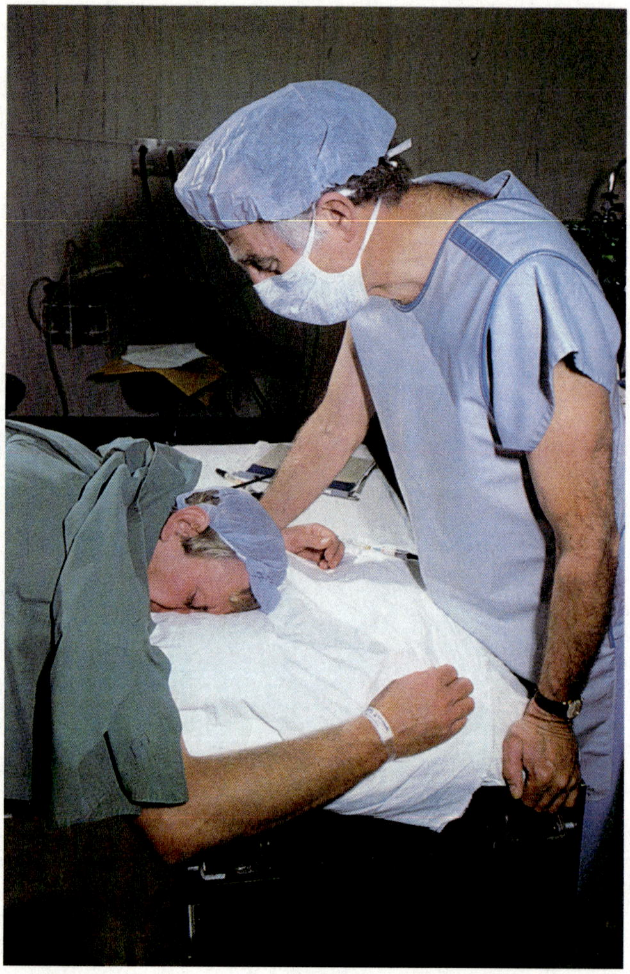

39

Application of dressing

40 Application of dressing. The points of needle penetration in the posterior midline area and in the lateral area have been covered by sterile dry dressings. These dry dressings are applied immediately after the needles are withdrawn.

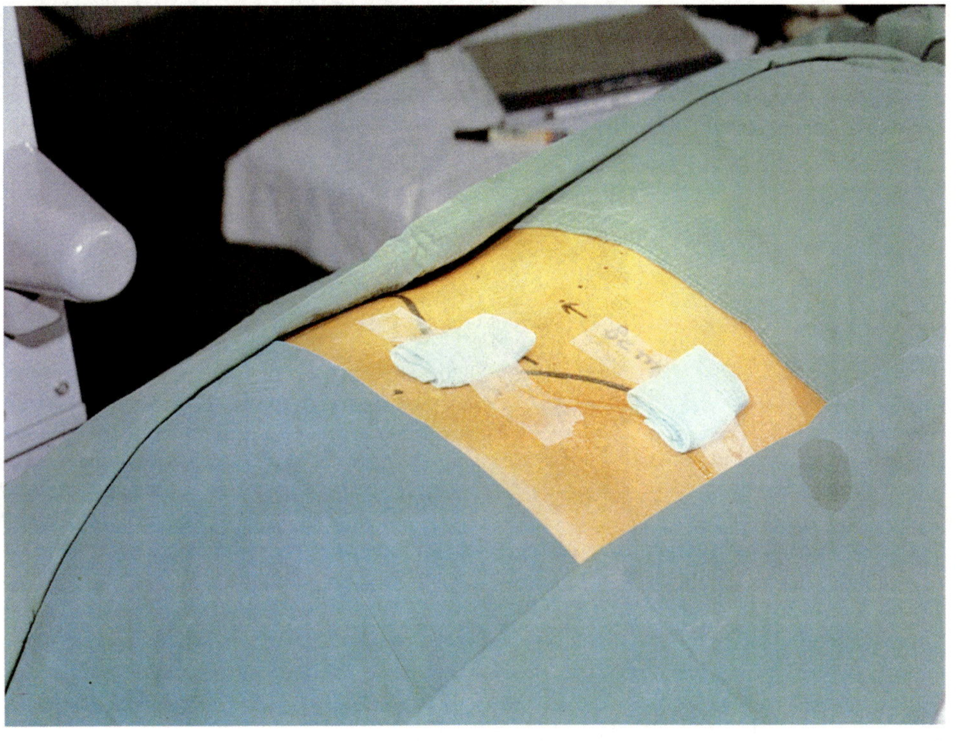

40

41 Return of patient to trolley after procedure completed. The patient is being rotated off the rest by lifting the handle. Note how easy it is to do this should it have to be done quickly, because, say, of anaphalactic shock.

41

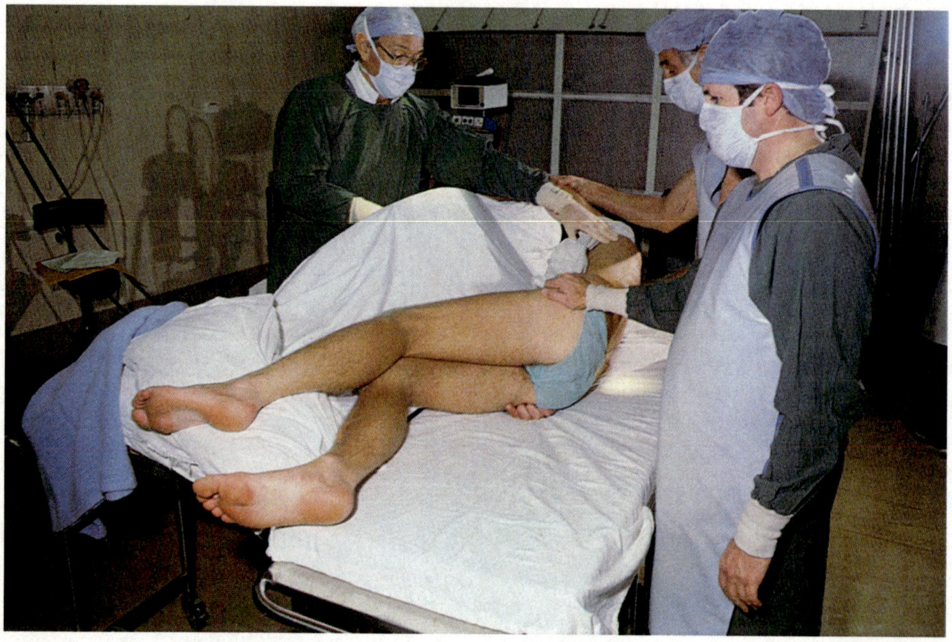

42 **Return of patient to trolley after procedure completed.** Note that the patient is rolled on to his back with the anaesthetist supporting his head and the radiographer helping to lower him on to the trolley.

42

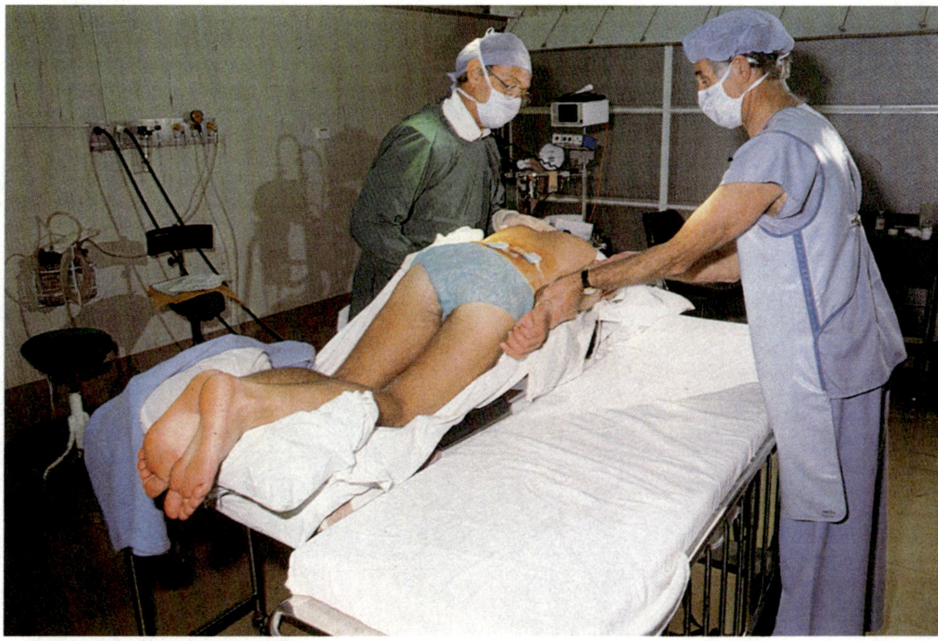

Manipulation of lumbar spine

43 Manipulation of lumbar spine. Supine patient awaiting manipulation of lumbar spine. In view of the great therapeutic value of spinal manipulation in the treatment of low back pain many surgeons take this opportunity to manipulate the spine with the patient asleep and relaxed under thiopentone anaesthetic. Here we see the pentothal sodium or thiopentone being administered intravenously by the anaesthetist.

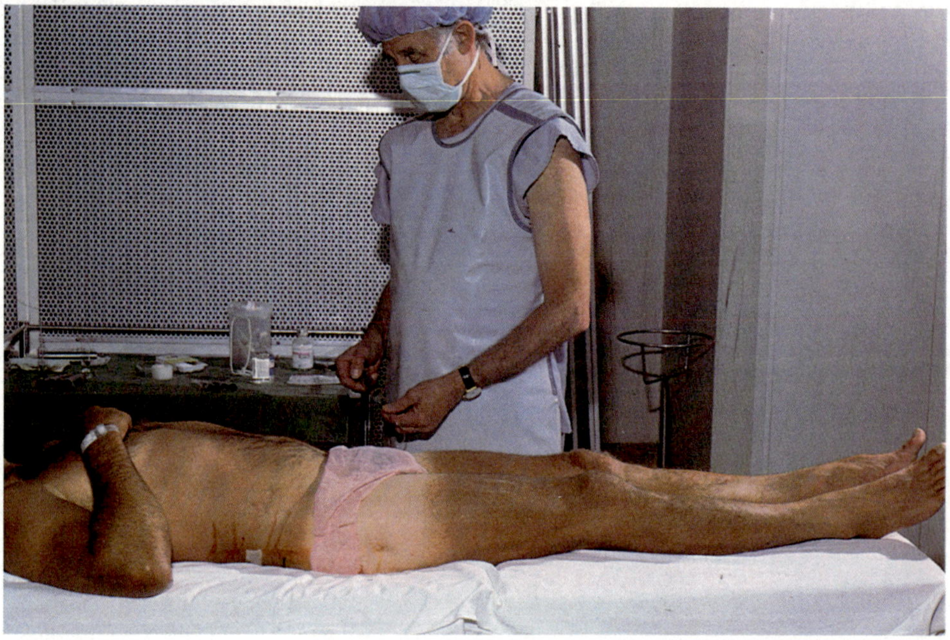

43

44 Flexing the lumbar spine. The first manoeuvre is to fully flex the lumbar spine by placing both flexed knees on the chest of the patient.

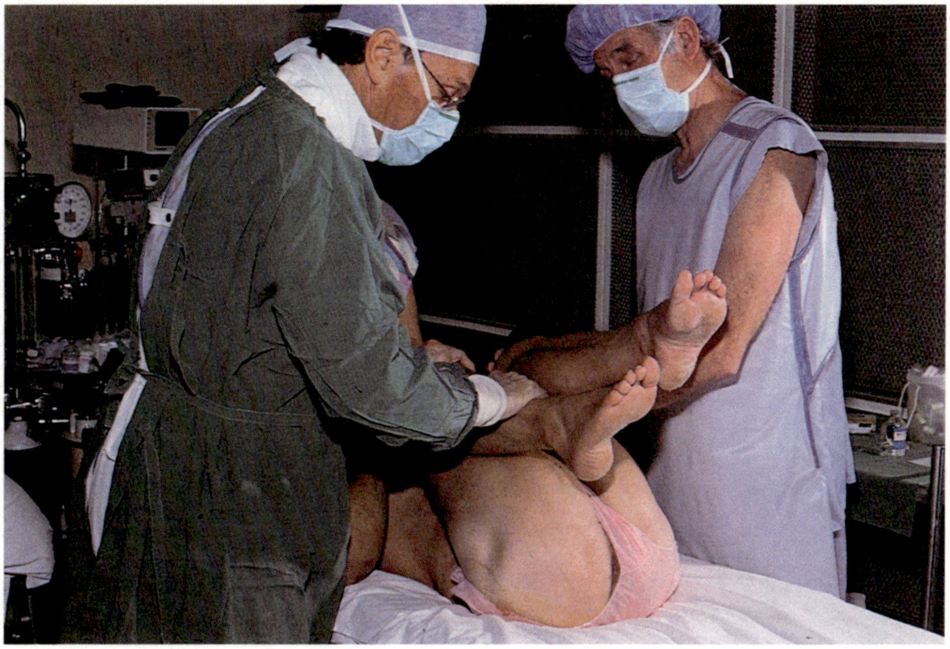

44

45 Rotation of pelvis to the right. Here the shoulders are held in the horizontal plane while the pelvis is rotated through 90 degrees to the right side by the two manipulators.

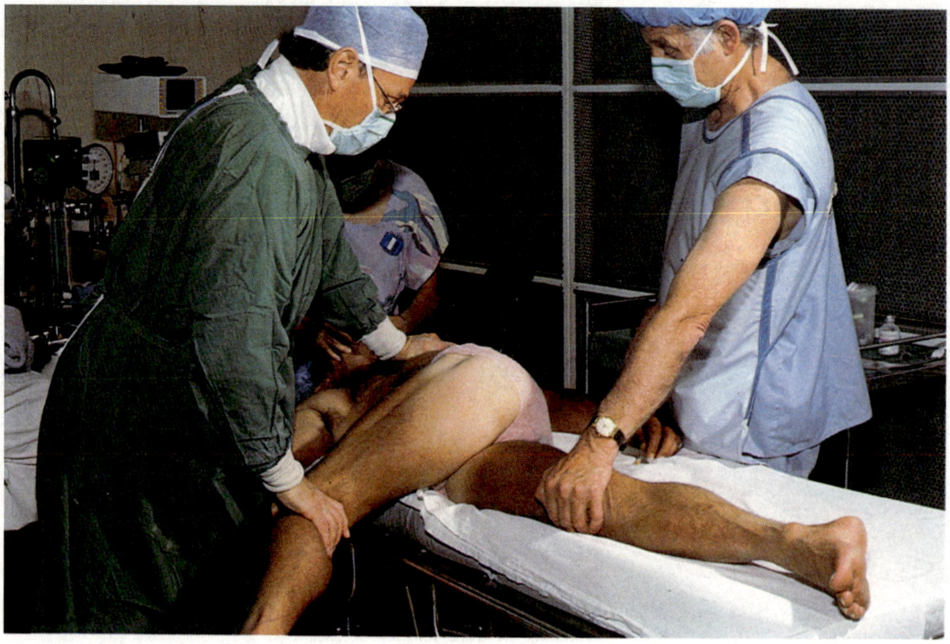

45

46 Rotation of pelvis to the left. With the shoulders pinned to the bed in the horizontal plane, the pelvis is rotated to the left through 90 degrees.

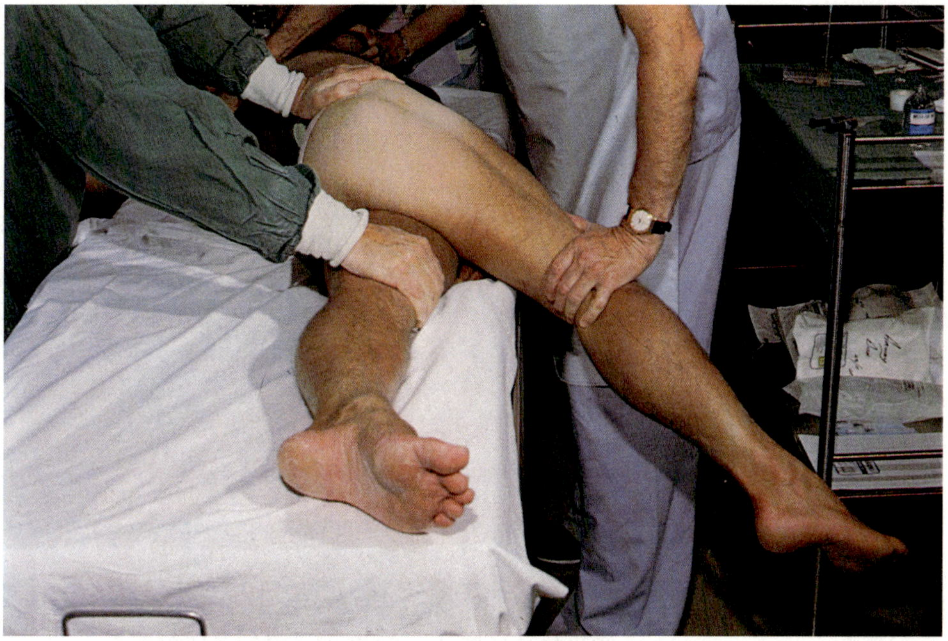

46

47 **Tilt of pelvis to the right.** With the torso held firmly the pelvis is rotated to the right thus opening the facet joints and intervertebral foramina on the left side of the lumbar spine.

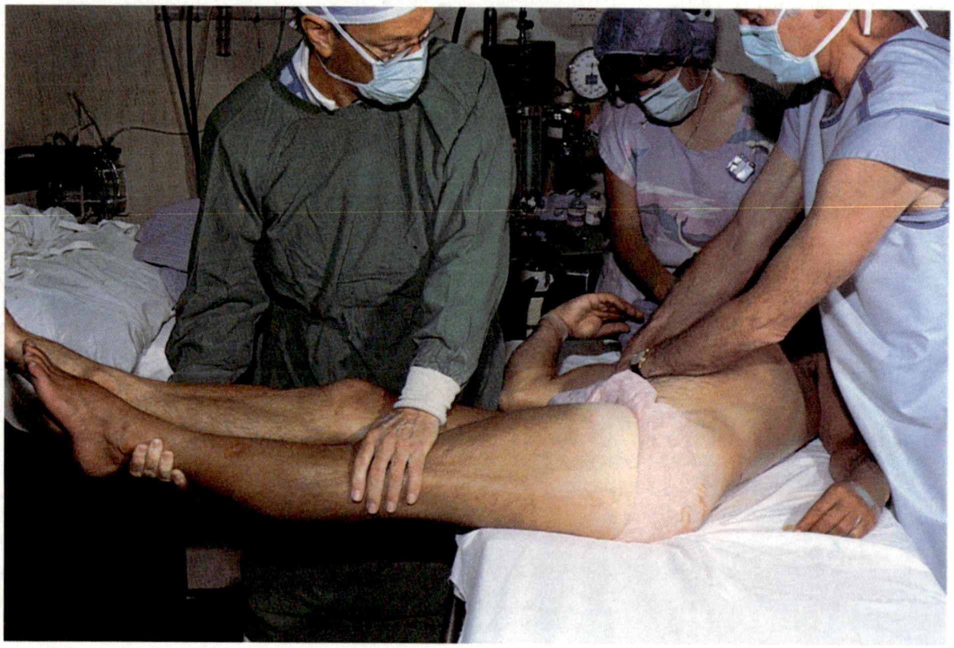

47

48 Tilt of pelvis to the left. Once again with the torso held firmly the pelvis is rotated to the left, thus opening up the facet joints and intervertebral foramina on the right side of the lumbar spine.

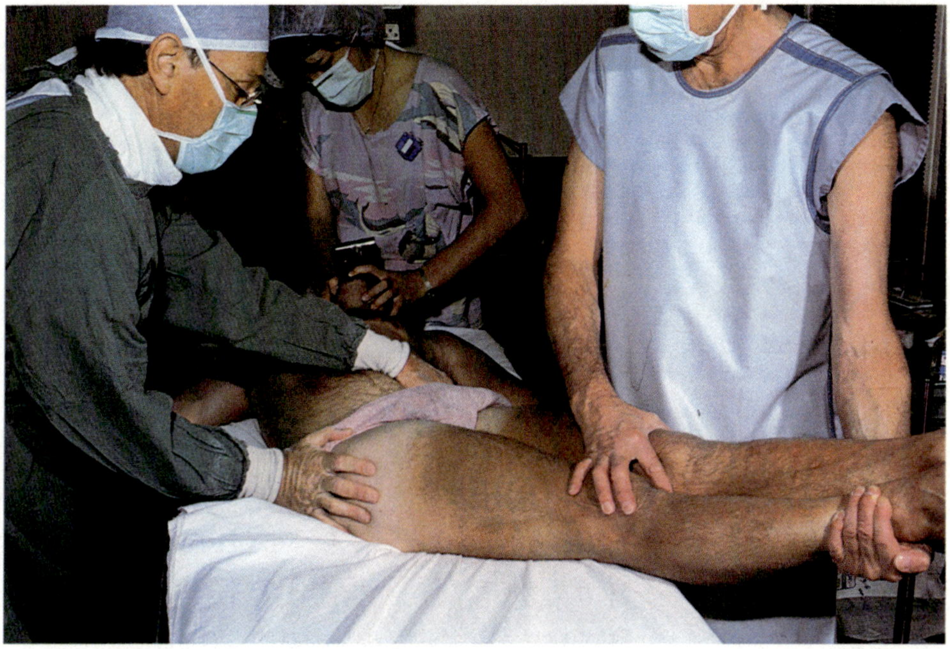

48

49 Extension of lumbar spine. With hands clasped behind the lumbar spine the manipulators lift the lumbar spine forward, thus exerting an extension force on this part of the spine.

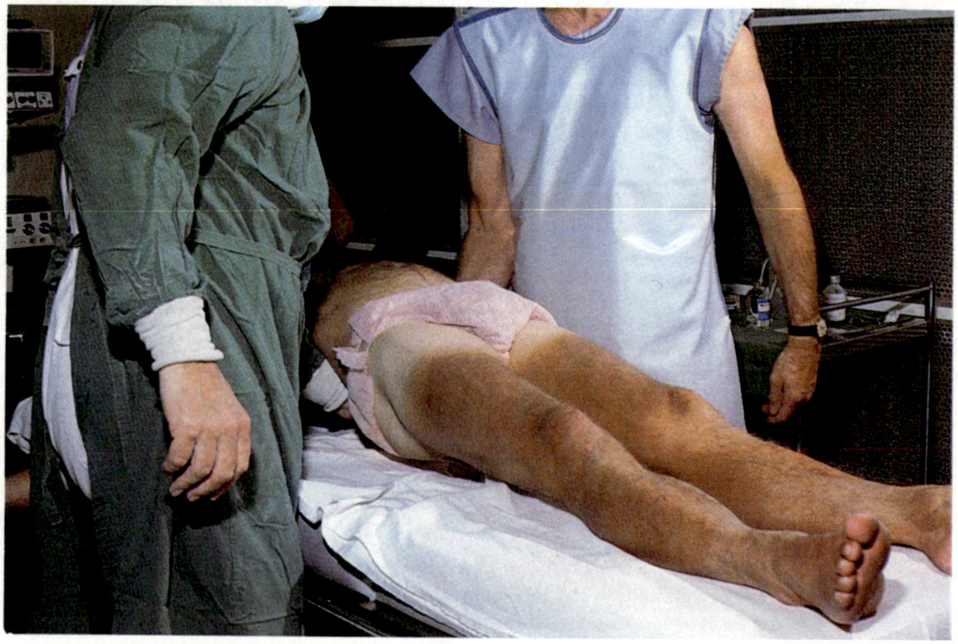

49

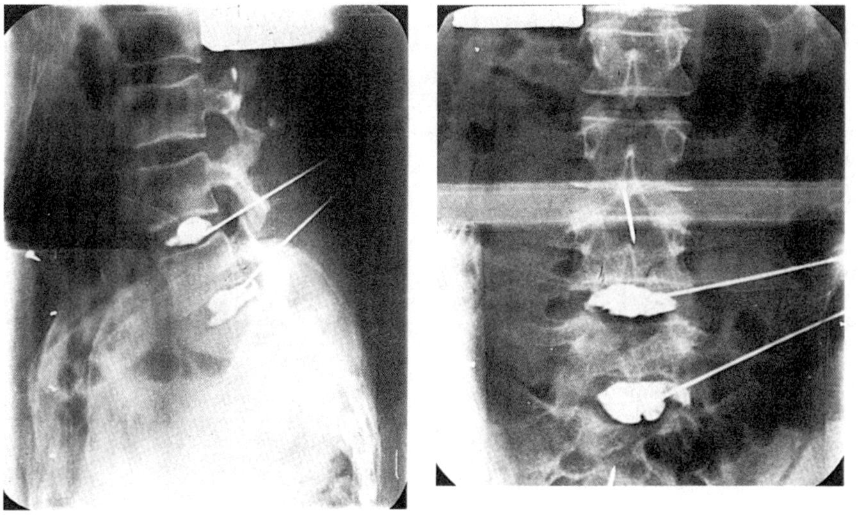

50

50 Lateral and anteroposterior xrays showing a discogram with a posterior protrusion at L-5.S-1 level. In the anteroposterior view it can be seen that the radio-opaque material is emerging through a defect in the annulus to the right side. The L-4-5 disc is normal in both views.

The varying patterns of normality

There are four basic types of normal discograms, which are (1) bilocular, (2) unilocular, (3) spherical, and (4) rectangular.

51 Anteroposterior and lateral view of the normal discogram known as the bilocular variety. Note that the radio-opaque material in the disc centre is in two globules, which are connected in the mid region. Note also that the annulus anteriorly and posteriorly is intact and that the cartilage plate through which nutrition passes to and from the disc is intact superiorly and inferiorly.

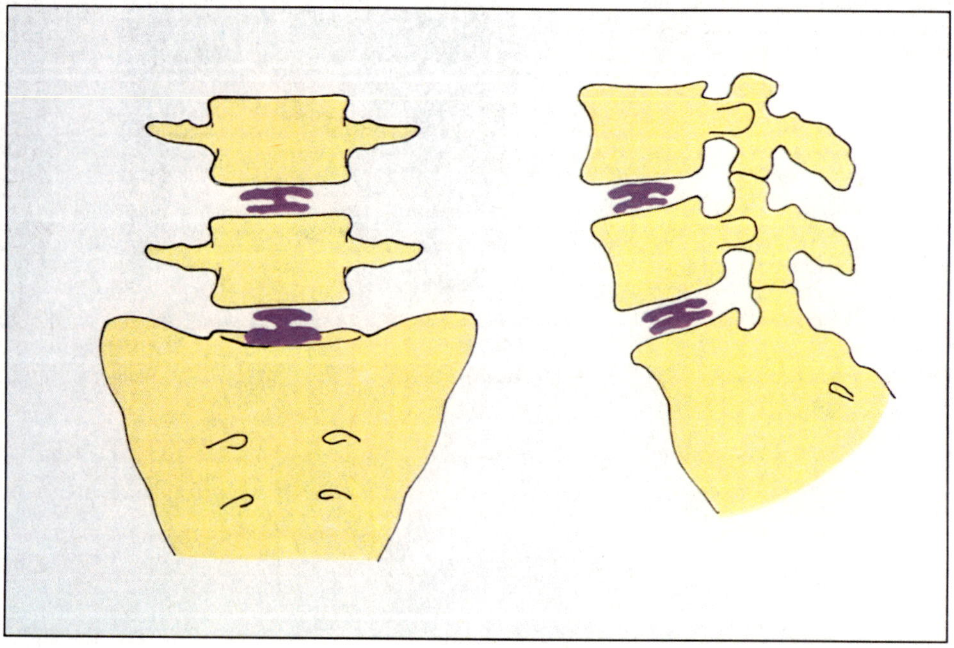

51

52 Normal discograms. An antero-posterior view on the left and a lateral view on the right showing a unilocular normal disc at L-4-5 level and a spherical normal disc at L-5.S-1 levels in both views.

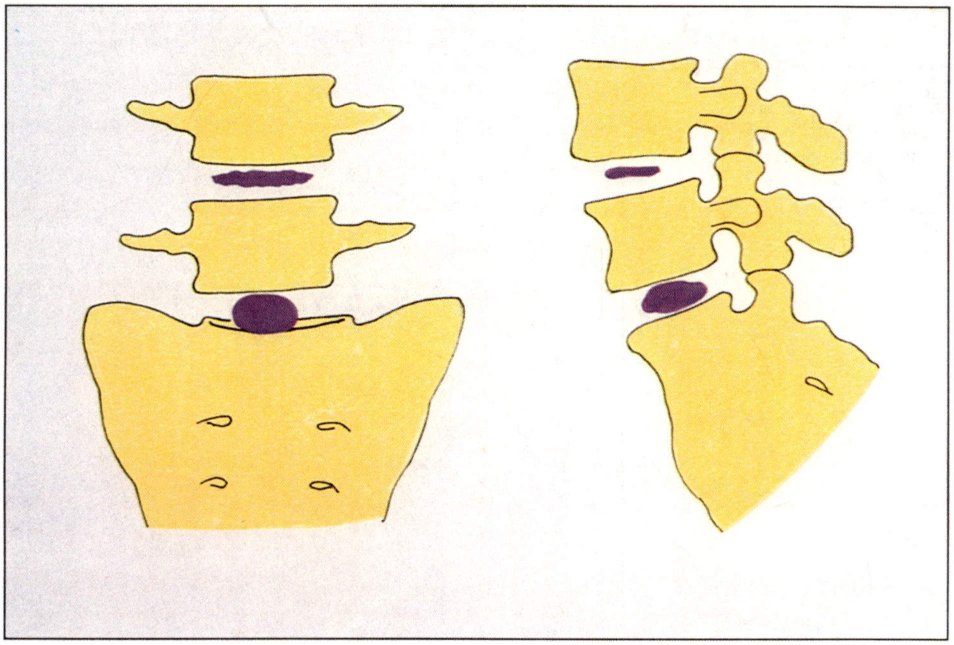

52

53 Normal discogram. An antero-posterior and lateral view of the rectangular type of normal discogram at L-5.S-1 level.

Note that in all four normal discograms the annulus fibrosus is intact around the nucleus pulposus superiorly and inferiorly and on both sides laterally. Above and below the nucleus pulposus is the intact cartilage plate.

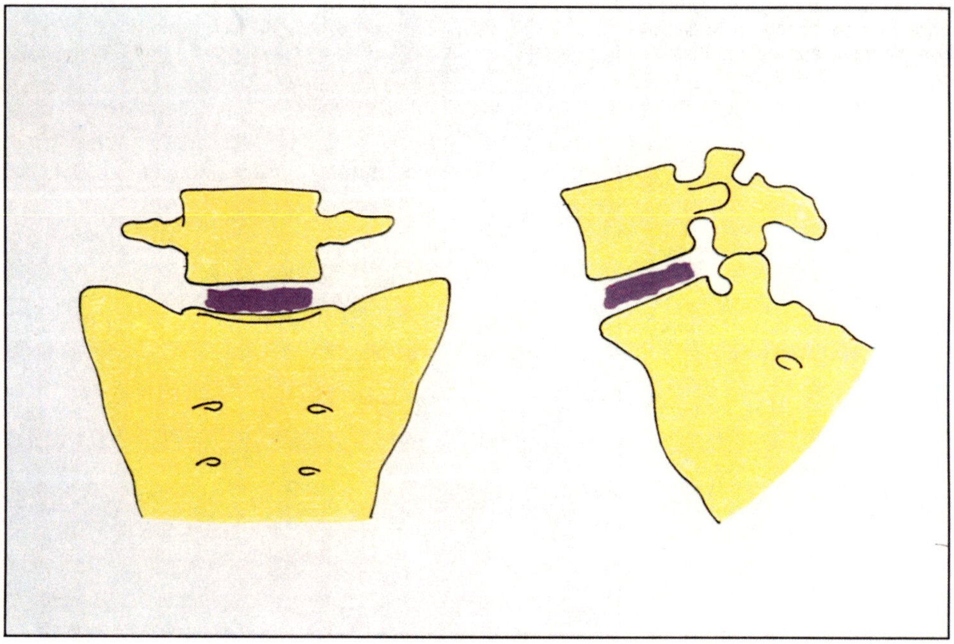

53

Discograms – The varying patterns of abnormality

These patterns may be summarised in the following diagrams.

54 Abnormal discograms. An antero-posterior view on the left with a normal L-4-5 disc and an extrusion at L-5.S-1 level. To the right we see normality again at L-4-5 and at L-5.S-1 the extrusion with escape of epidural dye. Extrusion with epidural escape of dye is usually associated with sequestration, which is defined as the escape of nuclear material into the spinal canal as a free fragment which may migrate to other locations.

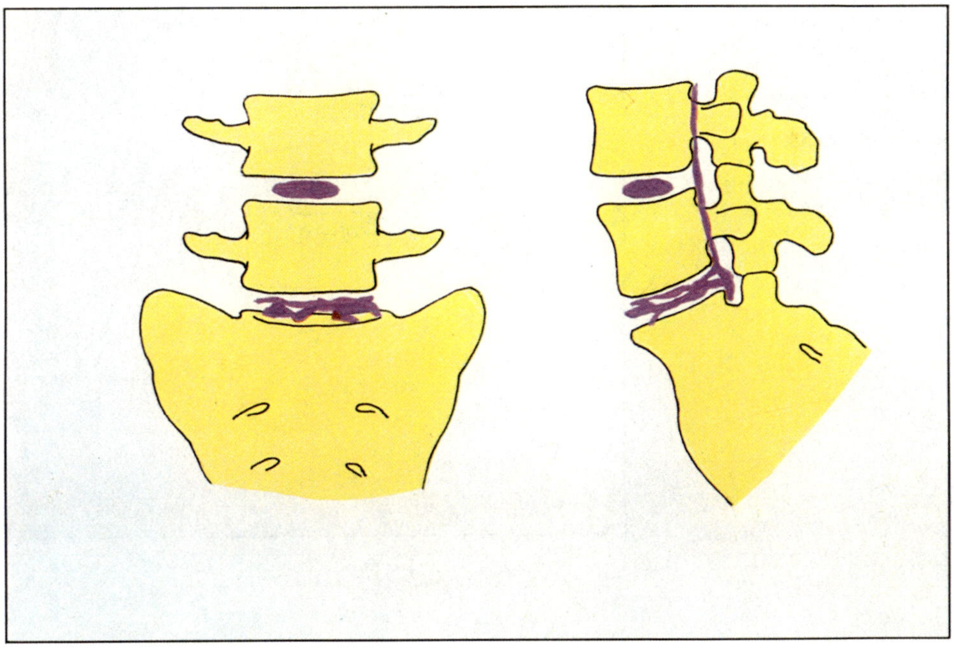

54

55 Abnormal discograms. The anteroposterior view on the left shows a lateral protrusion at L-4-5 level and a normal spherical disc at L-5.S-1. On the right hand side are a posterior protrusion at L-4-5 and a normal spherical disc at L-5.S-1. A protrusion is defined as the situation when the displaced material causes a discreet bulge in the annulus but no material escapes through the annular fibres.

55

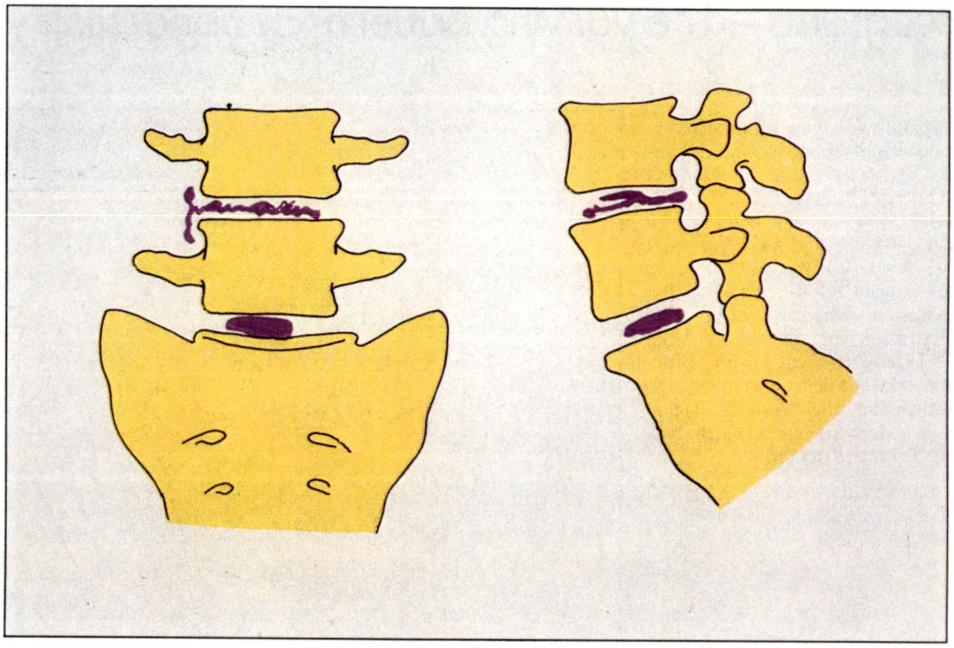

56 Abnormal discograms. On the left at L-4-5 level the normal bilocular disc is noted and at L-5.S-1 on the left hand side the contrast medium has been seen to be displaced into the body of the sacrum. On the right hand side of the picture we see at L-4-5 a bilocular normal disc and at L-5.S-1 the filling of a Schmorl's node into the sacrum. This Schmorl's node defect would probably be asymptomatic. It is usually painless and the phenomenon is called an intra-spongy nuclear herniation.

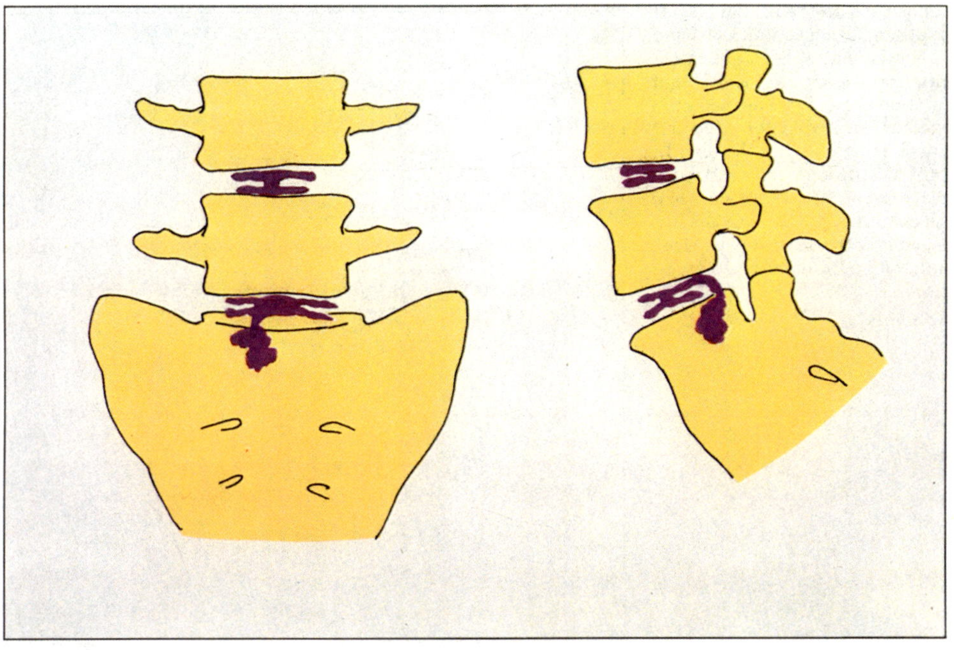

56

57 Abnormal discograms. On the left there is degeneration at both L-4-5 and L-5.S-1 levels and on the right side a posterior protrusion at L-4-5 and degeneration at L-5.S-1. Degeneration is defined as the loss of the structural and functional integrity of the disc. In cases of extrusion the displaced material presents in the spinal canal through disrupted fibres of the annulus but remains connected to material persisting within the disc.

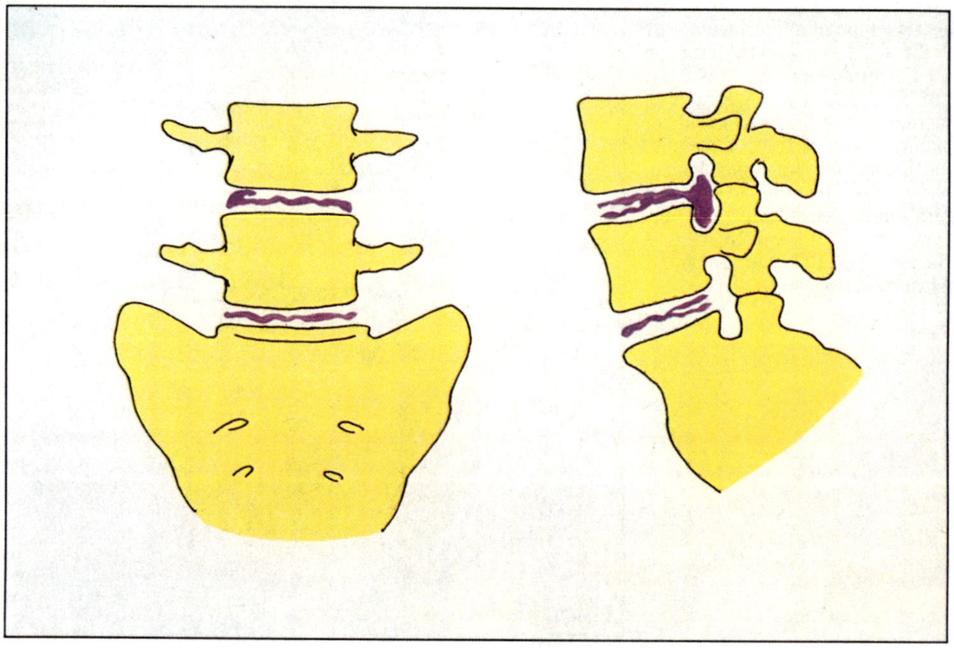
57

58 Abnormal discograms. On the left may be seen degeneration at L-4-5 and a normal bilocular disc at L-5.S-1. On the right there is degeneration at L-4-5 and normality at L-5.S-1.

58

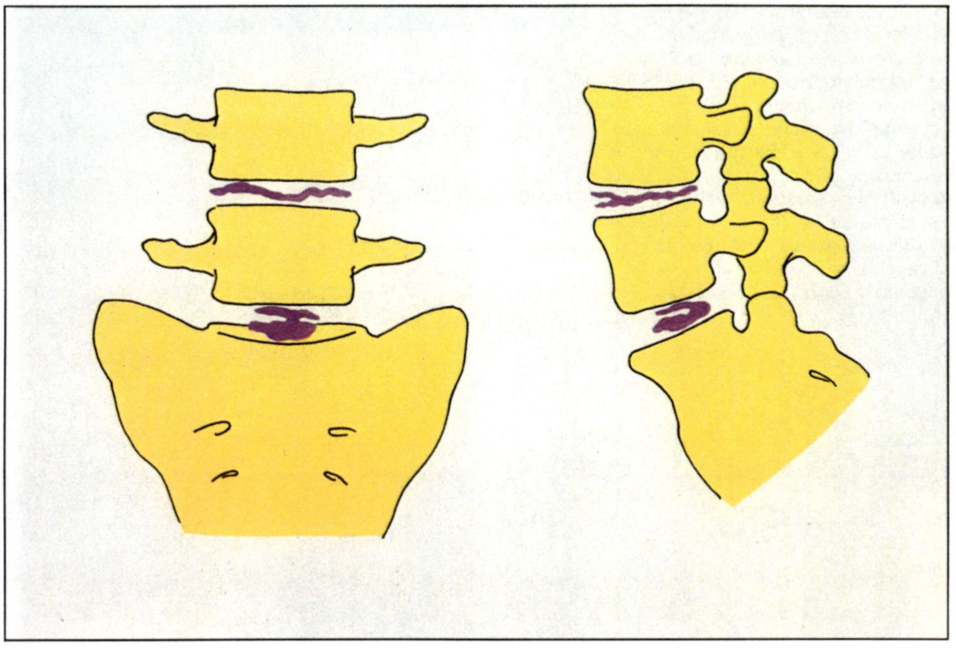

59 Abnormal discograms. On the left at L-4-5 level there is degeneration in the anteroposterior picture and a normal bilocular disc at L-5.S-1. On the right, however, there is extrusion with epidural dye escape at L-4-5 and normality at L-5.S-1. Extrusion with epidural escape of dye is usually associated with sequestration, which, as explained earlier, is defined as the escape of nuclear material into the spinal canal as a free fragment which may migrate to other localities.

59

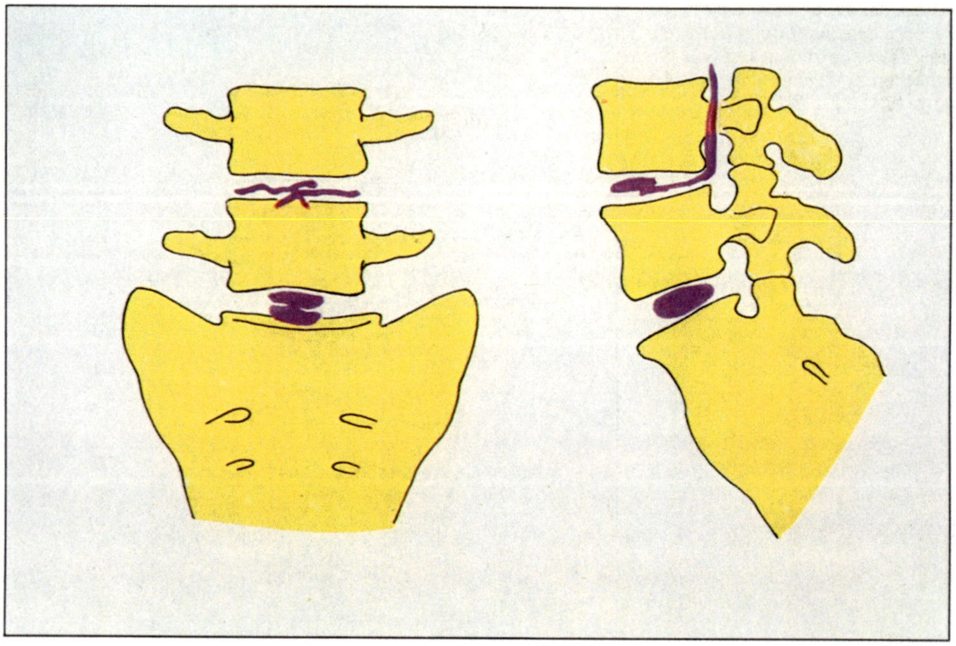

60 Abnormal discograms. On the left may be seen lateral protrusion at L-4-5 and a normal bilocular disc at L-5.S-1. On the right at L-4-5 level there is an anterior protrusion and a posterior protrusion at L-4-5 and at L-5.S-1 the disc is normal. There is marked degeneration at L-4-5. It is to be noted that an anterior protrusion is usually painless but the posterior protrusion at L-4-5 is probably associated with discogenic pain.

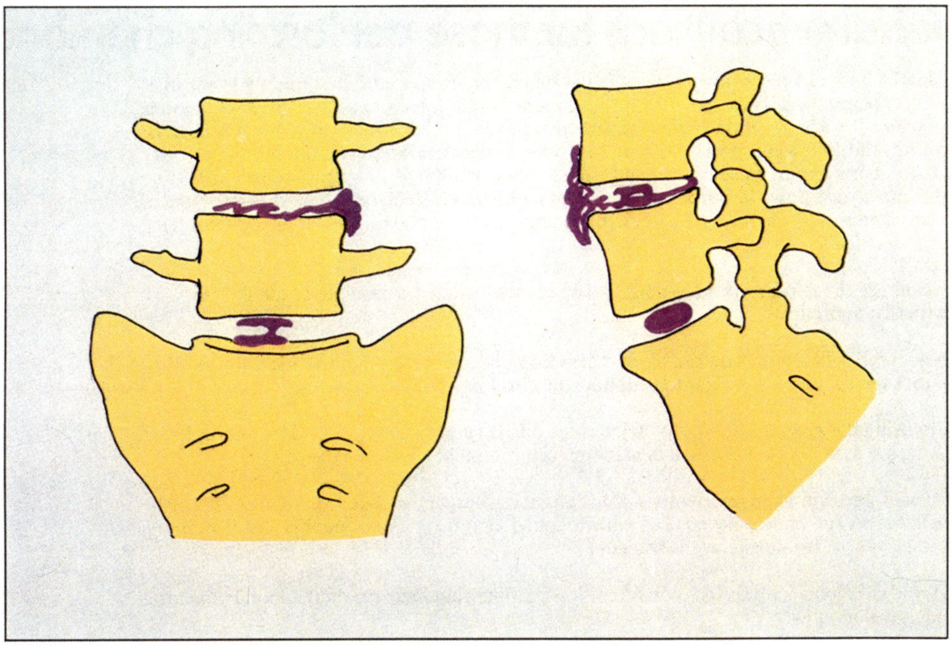

60

Special precautions for those performing chemonucleolysis

In a small number of cases, the presence in the subarachnoid space of the proteolytic enzymes used for chemonucleolysis may result in subarachnoid haemorrhage with very serious complications such as intracerebral haemorrhage or occlusion of spinal cord vessels. Therefore, the following special precautions to avoid penetration of the dural sac and entry into the subarachnoid space are recommended when lumbar discogram needles are to be placed into a disc for the purpose of performing chemonucleolysis – i.e. the injection of proteolytic enzymes (chymopapain or chymodiactin) into the disc centre for the relief of back pain and sciatica.

i) Never use the mid-line posterior approach because the needle must penetrate the dural sac with that approach.

ii) Select the needle insertion site 10 cm–12 cm from the mid-line rather than at the 8 cm mark – thus the needle is less likely to penetrate the dural sac.

iii) Try using the needle without the stylet as the disc is being approached, so that inadvertent dural sac penetration will result in a flow of cerebrospinal fluid from the needle.

iv) Always perform chemonucleolysis on a conscious, but well-sedated, patient so he or she will be aware of needle contact with a spinal nerve or cauda equina, so prompting redirection of the needle by the surgeon.

v) Avoid chemonucleolysis too soon after investigations that have resulted in dural puncture, e.g. myelography.

Conclusion

Lumbar discography is a reliable method of evaluating low back pain and radicular discomfort associated with herniation of the nucleus pulposus. It is an indispensable precursor to chemonucleolysis and is the most reliable preoperative diagnostic tool when, after failed conservative treatment, laminectomy and disc excision plus or minus fusion is being contemplated. From a diagnostic point of view it has proved more reliable than myelography, epidurography, and CAT scan.

It is well established that the myelogram at L-5.S-1 level will miss about 40 per cent of painful protruded or degenerated discs; the reason for this is simply that the gap between the dural sac and the disc in many patients is quite large and is usually filled with fat. A disc has to be extruded a good distance at L-5.S-1 level before it will be located by a myelogram. The epidurogram is technically quite difficult to perform in many cases. So far as the CAT scan is concerned I am in the process of doing a prospective study and it seems to date that many protrusions, extrusions, and sequestrations, seen clearly on the discogram, are missed by the CAT scan. Although, with the passage of time, one can expect improvements in CAT scanning hardware and expertise in its usage, the discogram has the advantage of offering the back pain sufferer some relief by virtue of the therapeutic agents that may be introduced into the disc through a centrally placed discogram needle. Ultimately, the CAT scanner may become so accurate in diagnosing disc herniation that the discogram needle will be used only for the introduction of therapeutic agents into the disc centre – thus avoiding the filling of the disc with Conray.

Index

All figures refer to page numbers.